A Color Atlas and Instruction Manual of Peripheral Blood Cell Morphology

A Color Atlas and Instruction Manual of Peripheral Blood Cell Morphology

Barbara H. O'Connor, M.S., S.H. (ASCP)

Teaching Supervisor, Clinical Hematology
Yale-New Haven Hospital
New Haven, Connecticut

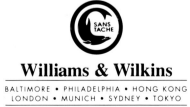

Williams & Wilkins

BALTIMORE • PHILADELPHIA • HONG KONG
LONDON • MUNICH • SYDNEY • TOKYO

A WAVERLY COMPANY

Copyright © 1984
Williams & Wilkins
428 E. Preston Street
Baltimore, MD 21202, U.S.A.

Made in the United States of America

Library of Congress Cataloging in Publication Data

O'Connor, Barbara H.
  A color atlas and instruction manual of peripheral blood cell morphology.

  Bibliography: p.
  Originally presented as the author's thesis (master's—Quinnipiac College, Hamden, Conn.)
  1. Blood cells—Atlases. I. Title. [DNLM: 1. Blood cells—Cytology—Atlases. 2. Hematologic diseases—Pathology—Atlases. QY 17 018c]
RB45.33   1982   616.1′50758′0222   81-10490
ISBN 0-683-06624-2

95 96 97   14 15

To my husband and my father
and
To my students, past, present, and future

FOREWORD

When thought of as a tissue, blood is one of the most easily biopsied in the body. More importantly, the distribution of the various cell types in a specimen as small as 1/1,000,000 of the total blood volume is highly representative of the blood as a whole. In contrast to biopsies of other tissues, sampling error is essentially nil. The broad clinical relevance of quantitative or qualitative deviations of blood cell types from normal coupled with the aesthetic beauty of stained blood film preparations probably explains why hematology atlases have been so popular in the past and remain so today.

This atlas was written from the viewpoint of one who has dealt with the practical problems involved in teaching morphologic hematology to medical residents, students, and technologists for more than two decades. It differs significantly from those currently available. The focus for this text has been directed towards detailing the morphologic characteristics that permit one to distinguish those cell types which are especially difficult to categorize. With great skill and using innovative approaches, Ms. O'Connor has carefully dissected those features which are most helpful in arriving at the most likely identification. Recognition criteria are presented descriptively in outline form and are accompanied by quality photomicrographs along with hand drawings meticulously detailed and carefully labeled.

Red cell morphology and estimation of platelet sufficiency are also uniquely treated. The author describes in very specific terms not only what to look for but also how to objectively quantitate abnormal red cell features and platelet numbers and provides specific guidelines for distinguishing normal from abnormal.

This work is obviously a labor of love written at a time when automation of the differential white blood count suggests a lessening demand for hematology technologists. One might question the need for another atlas. However, automation could well emphasize the need for competent morphologists. In the future it is likely that normal blood samples will be screened by machine as will many commonly occurring abnormal samples. However, those that remain will be problem specimens which contemporary electronics and automated instrumentation will be unable to cope with. Technologists and pathologists will deal primarily with such interesting abnormal preparations. Ms. O'Connor's atlas will help to ease the task, especially for beginning students in hematologic morphology. It represents a welcome addition to the library of hemato-morphologists.

Leonard S. Kaplow, M.D.
Director of Laboratories
Veterans Administration
Medical Center
West Haven, Connecticut
Professor of Pathology
and Medicine
Yale University
New Haven, Connecticut

PREFACE

The morphologic evaluation of cell type in Romanowsky-stained smears of peripheral blood presents continuing problems in hematology laboratories. This is quite evident in discussions, questions, survey results, and laboratory experiences. There is a desperate need for standardization in identifying cytomorphologic features and clarification of terms into one common definition for each cell type. Standardization is extremely important now when we are on the verge of having automated differential counters in our laboratories. Several authors and responsible committees have published position or clarification statements on the identification of specific cell forms. However, in the case of several ambiguous cells where there is a difference of opinion among master morphologists, the individual pathologist must choose the definition most compatible with his own experience and education, and have his laboratory staff perform blood cell identification in accordance with this definition.

Student morphologists, especially, have been greatly hampered by the lack of a good visual instruction manual that illustrates and describes each stage of maturation of every peripheral blood cell series. There is also a dearth of information about distinguishing morphologic features of cells in *dissimilar* cell lines with *similar* staining and physical characteristics, thus making identification difficult; *e.g.*, the promonocyte *versus* the myelocyte, the prorubricyte *versus* the plasma cell, etc.

It is not sufficient to tell the student or technologist, "You will learn it after a while by repetition and intuition." This leads to frustration and poor performance. It is essential to make consistent both observations and reporting for high quality results and interpretation.

I have been involved in teaching peripheral blood morphology since 1962 in two capacities. First, on a part-time basis, as the Section Chief in the hematology laboratory at Yale-New Haven Hospital, and then as the teaching supervisor in the same laboratory when student and technical staff increased to such proportions as to warrant a full-time instructor. My morphology instruction is aimed at medical technology students, freshman and sophomore medical students in the Yale School of Medicine, nursing practitioner Masters Degree candidates in the Yale School of Nursing, clinical pathology interns, and new employees to acquaint them with our differential methodology.

The instruction of this variety of individuals requires an organized study plan with a standardized nomenclature and set of definitions to establish precision on a day-to-day, person-to-person basis.

The first thing I had to do as a morphology instructor was to accumulate and maintain multiple stained smears of each blood dyscrasia. This can take months or years depending on the volume of and exposure to hematologic abnormalities at an institution. Second, a standardized procedure for the step-by-step performance of peripheral blood differentials, including nomenclature and descriptive definition of cell types, had to be written and made available to each student. Third, a set of color slides of each cell type and blood dyscrasia had to be obtained or photographed as a visual reinforcement to the written or oral instruction, especially when dealing with large groups at one time.

A major problem, however, has arisen because these teaching aids are separate and do not relate the written definition for a given cell or dyscrasia to an immediately accessible illustration. Available literature does not present a comparative pictorial study of the stages of development accompanied by explanatory text on the morphologically distinguishing features between these stages. Furthermore, enhanced understanding by the student would result if distinctive morphologic features were to be diagrammatically labeled and placed directly below each cell pictured. This is, in my opinion, the ideal arrangement for learning cellular morphology.

In its original form, this book was a thesis prepared for Quinnipiac College, in Hamden, Connecticut, as a requirement for the degree of Master of Health Science. In its current form, it represents my attempt to provide the student morphologist with a carefully organized pictorial, diagrammatic, and written instruction manual to assist in the learning of cellular characteristics and in the making of precise, accurate identification.

While students should keep in mind that no instruction manual can provide all the requisites for sophistication in morphologic identification, I sincerely hope it serves as a catalyst to stimulate them to acquire those attributes.

Barbara H. O'Connor

ACKNOWLEDGMENTS

Appreciation is expressed to the following individuals for their help and assistance in the completion of this project:

Dr. Leonard S. Kaplow, Dr. William R. Bronson, and Dr. Gokaldas C. Parikh who gave generously of their time and professional knowledge.

Dr. David Seligson, Director of Laboratories, Yale-New Haven Hospital, and Dr. Peter McPhedran, Director of Hematology Laboratory, Yale-New Haven Hospital, for providing the optimal laboratory environment which served as a catalyst for this paper.

Stanly S. Katz, Dean of Allied Health Programs, Quinnipiac College, who believed in the concept of this presentation.

Dr. Howard Pearson, Chief of Pediatrics, Yale-New Haven Hospital; Dr. Norma Granville, Director of Hematology Laboratory, St. Francis Hospital; Dr. William Bronson, Director of Hematology Laboratory, Hartford Hospital; Jean Raccio, Chief Technologist, St. Raphael's Hospital; Jeanne Raccio, William Jones, and Vera Kukil, for lending me their peripheral blood smears to photograph for this atlas.

Tom McCarthy, Ann Curley, Phill Simon, and Nathan Balducci, for the photographs in Chapter 3.

CONTENTS

LIST OF COLOR FIGURES

LIST OF TABLES

INTRODUCTION

It should be noted that the manual differential peripheral blood cell count procedure in Chapter 4 has been performed by the hematology laboratory staff at Yale-New Haven Hospital for the past 15 years and has been most effective in establishing precise and accurate differential examinations. Our laboratory is staffed by approximately 50 technologists who perform 250 manual differential peripheral blood cell counts daily. Because Yale-New Haven is a large referral center for the eastern part of the United States approximately one-third of these differential counts are abnormal. Therefore, it is extremely important to have a standardized differential procedure.

Wright's-stained peripheral blood films on glass slides were used, for the most part, as source material for the photographs in this volume. The exceptions are: 1) reticulocytes were stained with new methylene blue; 2) color prints in Chapter 3 are unstained peripheral blood smears; 3) the plasmacytic series was taken from Wright's-stained pleural fluid smears; and 4) the megaloblastic rubricytic series and the megakaryocyte are from Wright's-stained bone marrow preparations.

The photographs in this volume (with the exception of those in Chapter 3) were taken from a Kohler-illuminated Nikon microscope equipped with a Nikon Automatic Microflex Model AFM photographic attachment and using Kodak Ektachrome film (ASA64). The magnification index $\frac{1}{2}$ was set at ASA 100 with the D-ADJ knob set at $\frac{1}{3}$ under, to compensate for the speed of the film used. The shutter speed was set at $\frac{1}{8}$ second. The 100/115V transformer was set at 10. An 80B filter was placed in a holder directly under the microscope condenser lens and a didymium filter was placed directly over the light source. The microscope was equipped with 15× ocular lenses for all photographs. The 100× objective was used for all split-frame photographs, giving a total magnification of 1500×. Full-frame photographs were taken with either the 100×, 70×, 40×, or 10× objectives, giving total magnifications of 1500×, 1050×, 600×, or 150×, respectively; all magnifications are labeled throughout the text.

The photographs in Chapter 3 were taken by the x-ray photography department at Yale-New Haven Hospital with a Besler TOPCON 55 mm lens camera equipped with an 81A magenta filter and 20M filter and illuminated by a fluorescent light box. Kodak Ektachrome E-4 film was used.

Chapter 1

The Functions of the Peripheral Blood Examination

The four important functions of the peripheral blood examination are:
1. To provide information for diagnosis.
2. To provide data for the selection of further pertinent tests to establish a diagnosis.[77]
3. As a guide to therapy.
4. As an indicator of harmful effects of chemotherapy and radiotherapy.[164]

Chapter 2

Proper Peripheral Blood Smear Preparation

Description of a Properly Prepared Slide

1. A smooth even surface, free from ridges, waves, and holes.[77]
2. A film spread that does not involve the edges of the slide or coverslip (manual methodologies).[77]
3. A film spread that consists of a monocellular layer over a large slide area (automatic methodologies).[123]
4. Leukocytes and erythrocytes should not touch or overlap and should be optimally separated unless agglutination is a symptom of a physiological condition for that specimen.[123]
5. The preparation method should not only treat the blood gently enough to retain the cell morphology, but should assure that observed traits are not artefacts of the technique.[123]
6. The cell distribution should be statistically uniform over the total slide area and should accurately reflect the whole blood volume distribution to ensure that the patient's condition is accurately determined.[123]

Prerequisites for Proper Peripheral Blood Smear Preparation

1. *Perfectly clean* frosted edge slides or coverslips.
2. 2–3 mm blood drop for optimal consistency.
3. Quick spreading of blood drop.
4. Rapid drying of smear to avoid contraction or artefacts.[44]
5. Proper placement of blood drop
   a. *Slide*: *manual method*—drop should be placed ½ inch from frosted edge for push and spread slide techniques.
      Slide: *automatic method*—blood drop should be placed on center of slide.
   b. *Coverslip*: drop should be placed "bull's eye" center of the 22 mm square.[44]
6. Differential smears should be made immediately when possible and no later than 3 hours after sample collection for good preservation of cellular morphology. Degenerative changes are minimal in EDTA-anticoagulated blood specimens performed within 1 hour of collection.[40]

Chapter 3

Techniques of Peripheral Blood Smear Preparation

Automated peripheral blood cell differential systems are currently under development and some limited white blood cell differential systems are in use in several laboratories throughout the country. In order to take maximum advantage of these automated blood differential systems, a technique or device for producing monolayers of uniformly stained peripheral blood slides is most desirable. The conventional methods of wedge or spread slide and coverslip preparations of blood films were found to have serious shortcomings when viewed as part of an overall white cell differential system. The primary deficiency in these methodologies is that operator skill influences the quality of the blood film, the number of ruptured or distorted cells, and the size and shape of the "good" area.[150]

The *wedge slide* technique is described by Wintrobe as producing an excellent smear for morphologic studies. However, it has several disadvantages: 1) it is difficult to teach to new personnel and students; 2) the cellular distribution is non-uniform throughout the film with the large leukocytes (polymorphonuclear leukocytes and monocytes) being pulled to the edge and the lymphocytes remaining scattered throughout the smear; and 3) small crowded red blood cells occur at the thick edge and large flat red blood cells without central pallor occur at the feathered edge.[187]

The *spread slide* technique was instituted in our laboratory at Yale-New Haven Hospital in the mid-1960's shortly after we purchased an Ames Hema-Tek Stainer to stain our peripheral blood films when blood samples became too voluminous to maintain manual staining of coverslip smears. We discovered that the Ames Hema-Tek Stainer did not stain the last 1/4 inch of the slide on each end. In order to establish uniform staining results for our peripheral blood films I decided to experiment and applied the spread technique of the coverslip methodology to 3 inch by 1 inch glass slides. I discovered that the blood print could be kept in the center of the slide and, at the same time, a feathered edge was achieved on both ends of the smeared blood thus eliminating the unstained edge effect and providing a larger "good" area of blood sample to evaluate for differential examination in comparison to the wedge slide and coverslip techniques. If a 2–3 mm drop of blood was used for the peripheral smear, then the blood remained spread on the bottom slide with no grossly visible blood retained on the top slide. Thus, it could be used on the uncontaminated side for the subsequent blood film, eliminating the wastage of any slides. A study of cellular distribution on the spread slide technique has not been conducted to my knowledge.

Examination of the literature on the *coverslip* blood film preparation seems to indicate that there is some disagreement as to the quality of this type of film. MacGregor *et al.*[113] note that "films on coverslips do not offer regularity of distribution of the leukocytes which can be obtained in slide films." Boveri[23] compared coverslip and wedge slide preparations to Burker chamber counts and concluded that the coverslip was the method of choice for it gave a differential count that correctly represented the relative proportions of the different types of white blood cells in the original drop of blood.[23] However, 1) the coverslip method is very difficult to teach and to master, 2) it does not lend itself to automated staining systems, and 3) the coverslip must be mounted on a glass slide which requires more time and expense than the slide techniques.

Now with the advent of automated peripheral blood differential systems, various types of automated slide spinners are being manufactured to produce large area monolayer blood films which are uniform in distribution of the various cell types. The use of spinners for peripheral blood smear preparation was first suggested by Preston and Ingram.[139] The most striking feature of the spun smears has been the high degree of uniformity over the entire slide surface. Platelets and leukocytes are almost always monodispersed on the spun smears which is the optimal presentation for numerical estimation and cellular identification. The edge effect seen in coverslip and wedge slide preparations, where the heavier cell, the monocyte, is found in higher concentrations at the periphery of the smear, is not seen on automatically spun smears. The problem of how to deal with blood samples of varying viscosity had to be resolved to achieve good red blood cell presentation on spun smears. Please refer to page 12 for a further discussion of the types of automatic slide devices or spinners and their resolution of the blood viscosity problem.

Push Slide Technique or Wedge Slide Technique

1. Hold a 1 inch by 3 inch glass slide by the narrow side between the thumb and forefinger of the left hand and place a 2–3 mm drop of blood approximately ¼ inch from the frosted area of the glass slide with a wooden applicator stick which you hold between the thumb and forefinger of the right hand.
2. Place the slide containing the blood droplet on a flat surface (usually the counter top of the laboratory bench) and hold firmly by the narrow side of the slide between the thumb and forefinger of the left hand at the end farthest from the drop of blood.
3. Grasp a second slide (the spreader slide) between the thumb and forefinger of the right hand.[31]
4. Place this spreader slide on the lower slide in front of the blood droplet and pull back until it touches the drop.[125]

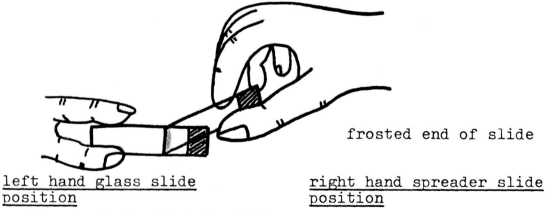

frosted end of slide

<u>left hand glass slide</u>
<u>position</u>

<u>right hand spreader slide</u>
<u>position</u>

Figure 3.1.   Position of left-hand and right-hand glass slides for push slide technique or wedge slide technique of peripheral blood smear preparation.

5. Allow blood to spread by capillary attraction almost to the edge of the slide.[125]
6. Push the spreader slide forward at approximately a 30° angle using a rapid, even motion. The weight of the slide should be the only pressure applied.[125]

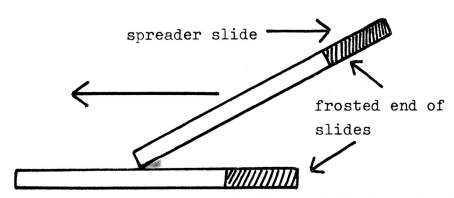

Figure 3.2. Direction of movement of spreader slide to make blood smear. *Note:* The thickness of the spread is influenced by: 1) angle of spreader slide (the greater the angle, the thicker and shorter the blood film, 2) size of blood droplet, and 3) speed of spreading.

A good slide preparation should be thick at one end and thin at the opposite end. This thin area, in which red blood cells are evenly dispersed, should be at least 2 cm long.[125] The blood film should occupy the central portion of the slide and should be margin-free on all sides.

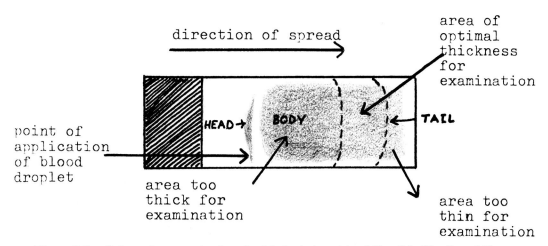

Figure 3.3. Schematic example of push slide technique blood film. (Modification of Figure 12 in Dacie, J.V. and Lewis, S.M. *Practical Hematology*, 3rd ed. Grune & Stratton, Inc., New York, 1968, p. 55.)[40]

Caution: In the push slide technique of blood smear preparation, larger leukocytes such as the monocyte and the neutrophil, will be higher at the periphery of the blood film than in the body of the blood film and lymphocytes will be higher in the body of the blood film and lower at the periphery of the blood film.[40]

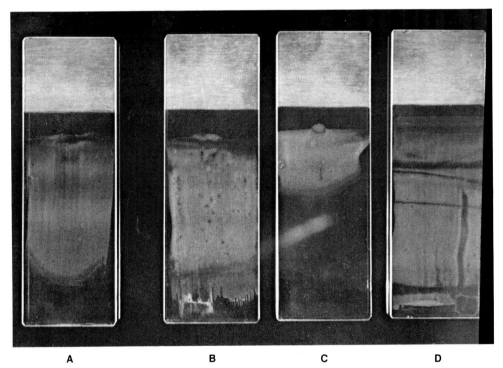

Figure 3.4.   Optimal and poor examples of push slide technique or wedge slide technique. *A.* Example of optimal preparation. *B.* Poor example with small voids of blood due to greasy film on slide and too large a droplet of blood causing excess thickness. *C.* Poor example resulting from small droplet of blood being spread too rapidly. *D.* Poor example with jerks and ridges due to uneven pressure while preparing or to use of unclean slides.

Spread Slide Technique

1. Pick up a 1 inch by 3 inch frosted glass slide and hold it at the frosted edge between the thumb and forefinger of the left hand. This leaves the right hand free to place a 2–3 mm droplet of blood with a wooden applicator stick on the top of this slide approximately ¼ inch from the frosted area margin.
2. Pick up a second 1 inch by 3 inch glass slide with the thumb and forefinger of the right hand at the frosted edge of the slide.

3. Gently place the slide held in the right hand over the slide held in the left hand so that the right hand slide extends ½ inch past the blood droplet.

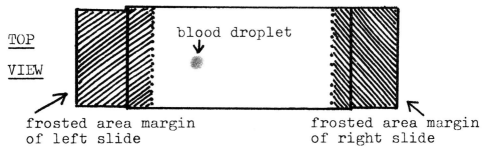

Figure. 3.5. Position of left-hand and right-hand slides for spread slide technique of peripheral blood smear preparation.

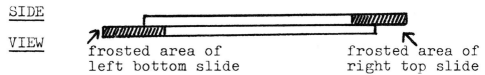

Figure 3.6 Side view of left-hand and right-hand slides for spread slide technique of peripheral blood smear preparation.

4. Allow a few seconds for spreading of the blood droplet and before it is completed, separate the two glass slides by a rapid but steady absolutely horizontal, lateral pull. There should be no lifting of either slide during the process.

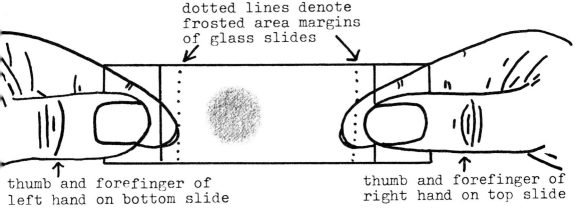

Figure 3.7. Position of left-hand and right-hand glass slides for spread slide technique of peripheral blood smear preparation.

5. The optimal blood smear preparation should exhibit a feathered effect at each end of spread blood droplet and the sides should be free of slide margins as schematically diagrammed below.

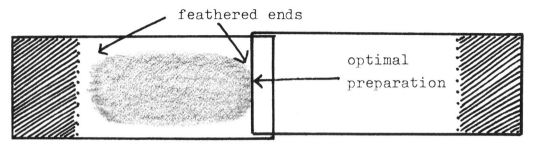

Figure 3.8. Schematic example of spread slide technique blood film.

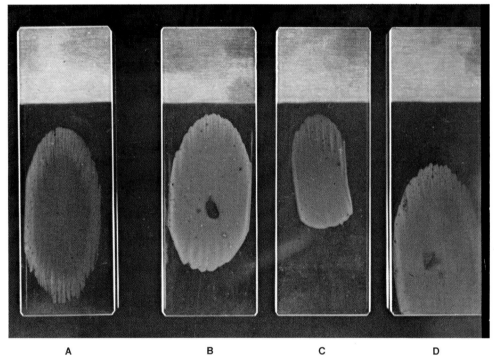

Figure 3.9. Optimal and poor examples of spread slide technique. *A.* Example of optimal preparation. *B.* Poor example with excess thickness due to too large a blood droplet. Small circular void of blood in this smear is due to either unclean area of slide or improper placement of top slide on blood droplet on bottom slide causing an air bubble during spreading. *C.* Poor example resulting from blood droplet being spread too rapidly. *D.* Poor example resulting from improper placement of blood droplet resulting in partial cutoff of smear.

Coverslip Technique

1. Pick up a 22 mm by 22 mm no. 1 coverslip by two adjacent corners between the thumb and index finger of the right hand. This leaves the left hand free to regulate the size of the droplet of blood (2–3 mm in diameter) to be picked up from the fingerstick puncture.[31]
2. The coverslip should be held just above the capillary blood droplet to allow the blood to reach the coverslip by capillary attraction and thereby avoid touching the skin.[31]
3. Pick up a second coverslip with the left hand and hold by one corner between the

thumb and index finger so that it forms a triangle while the coverslip in the right is held between the thumb and index finger so it forms a square.

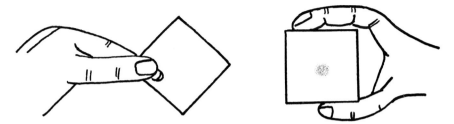

Figure 3.10. Position of left-hand and right-hand coverslips for peripheral blood smear preparation.

4. Gently place the coverslip held in the right hand over the coverslip held in the left hand so that the two superimposed coverlips form an octagon.[31]

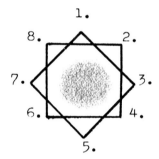

Figure 3.11. The octagonal appearance of superimposed coverslips.

5. Allow a few seconds for spreading of the blood droplet to occur and before it is completed the two coverslips are separated by a rapid, but steady absolutely horizontal, lateral pull. There should be no lifting of either coverslip during the process.[31] If the coverslips are not drawn in a strictly horizontal direction, an even distribution of cells will not occur and a jerk mark in the corner of the blood smear will result.

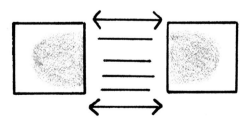

Figure 3.12. Appearance of completed horizontal, lateral pull of both coverslips. *Note:* It is imperative that paired coverslips on the same slide be derived from the same drop of blood for accurate distribution of cells.

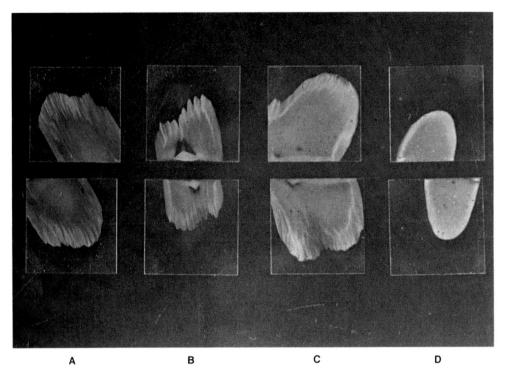

A   B   C   D

Figure 3.13. Optimal and poor examples of coverslip technique. *A.* Example of optimal preparation. *B.* Poor example with "jerk" mark due to lifting up of coverslip and catching point of slip as separation occurs. Coverslips must be kept perfectly level and slowly traverse each other during preparation. *C.* Poor example resulting in excess thickness due to too large a blood droplet. *D.* Poor example resulting from small blood droplet being pulled too rapidly.

Automatic Slide Spinner Technique

Various automatic devices or spinners have been developed for the preparation of peripheral blood smears for use with the new automated differential systems.

One such automatic device is Hemaprep which is manufactured by the Geometric Data Corporation and simulates the manual slide technique but fixes the angle of a spreader glass (rather than a slide) while allowing the operator to select a variety of predetermined speeds for drawing blood across the slide. A mechanical means is used to move the slide instead of moving the spreader manually.[180]

Automatic spinners hold a 3 inch by 1 inch microscope slide on a platen in a horizontal plane perpendicular to the shaft of the motor. A small pool of blood is deposited on the middle of the slide. Surface tension holds the blood in place until the lid of the spinner is closed which activates the motor to produce rapid acceleration to the desired spin speed and a rapid stop after the desired spin time.[123]

Bacus showed that it was important to spin blood samples for a time proportional to the red blood cell concentration.[7] He found that the hematocrit, the volume percentage of erythrocytes in whole blood, could be used as a criterion to adequately predetermine the spinning time for consistent cell separation. Using a motor with rapid acceleration and deceleration, the time range for spinning blood samples for hematocrit values between 10% and 60% was found to vary from 0.5 to 2.5 seconds. In order to avoid the need for a hematocrit determination prior to making each blood film, a photodetector was developed. This device optically senses the concentration of cells in the bulk volume of undiluted whole blood as spinning proceeds and the cells spread apart. When cells are sufficiently spaced, spinning is stopped. This is the principle of action of the LARC automatic spinner manufactured by Corning Medical Glass Works, Medford, MA.[7]

Nourbakhsh *et al.*[130] conducted their studies on automatic spinners utilizing the Model 90 Unismear Spinner (Coleman Division of Perkin-Elmer Corporation, Maywood, IL) and an early prototype of the Model 301 Spinner (Perkin-Elmer Corporation, Norwalk, CT).[130] The model 301 Spinner is capable of diluting the whole blood samples and automatically pipetting the sample on the slide as well as providing a temperature-controlled environment for optimal cellular separation. Nourbakhsh *et al.*[130] prepared their blood smears on the above mentioned spinners which rotate with a fixed velocity for a fixed time. All K_3EDTA-anticoagulated whole blood samples that they used for spun smears were first diluted with a fixed ratio of 2 parts blood to 1 part diluent (isotonic buffered saline solution). The diluting of whold blood samples prior to blood smear preparation excludes carryover by cleansing the inside of the pipettor after each sampling and reduces the viscosity of the blood to facilitate spinning. If the dilution step is omitted, blood samples which vary widely in their viscosity due to their plasma protein content and their hematocrit could not be spun at a single setting for spinning time and velocity and achieve good representative red blood cell morphology in nearly all of these blood specimens.[130]

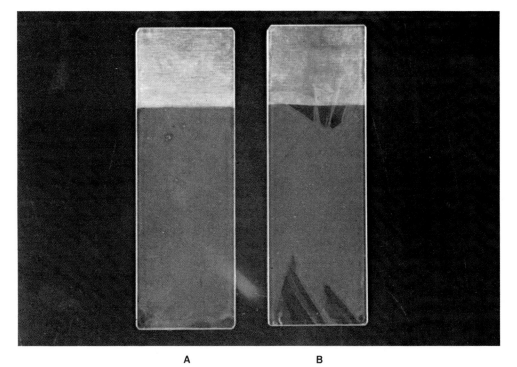

A   B

Figure 3.14.   Optimal and poor examples of automatic slide spinner technique. *A*. Example of optimal preparation. *B*. Poor example which could only occur if the individual completely ignores instructions as to the size of the blood droplet and the speed and time settings designated for use with the spinner.

Chapter 4

The Peripheral Blood Differential Cell Count

Problems Associated with Wright's Stain

Wright's stain, a Romanowsky-type blood stain, is used extensively in the hematology laboratory for the routine staining of peripheral blood smears. In 1890, Romanowsky discovered that a purplish-red stain, methylene azure, which is an oxidation product of methylene blue, is produced when old moldy methylene blue is mixed with eosin. In 1891, Malachowski demonstrated that this new metachromatic stain could be consistently obtained by alkalinizing methylene blue in Na_2HCO_3 solution and subsequently adding eosin, thus making it unnecessary for mold formation to occur. This dye may be purchased as a powder which is then dissolved in methyl alcohol or a ready-made solution may be obtained.[186]

One major problem in using Romanowsky-type blood stains is the large variation in staining properties between the same stain type provided by different suppliers and between different batches from the same suppliers. The major causes of component variations in Wright's stain include[111]: 1) the unavailability of pure dyes used in stain construction; 2) the lack of control in polychroming these dyes, and the instability of thiazine dyes in solution due to loss of methanol from the stain because of evaporation and acquisition of water vapor by the hygroscopic absolute methanol in the stain; and 3) the lack of an adequate method for separating and quantitating individual stain components.

Small variations in color and intensity of stained leukocytes may be tolerated when the stain is observed by a highly trained technologist, since classification decisions are made on the basis of information gathered over the entire visible spectrum.

With the advent of automated blood differential analyzers which utilize color and pattern recognition techniques for the identification of stained leukocytes, a consistently reliable Wright's staining reaction has become of paramount importance. To ensure minimal compositional variation in stain for the new automated methodology, unique manufacturing procedures have been developed and chromatographic assays have been introduced for quantitative quality control.[111]

This peripheral blood cell differential procedure has been performed in the Clinical Hematology Laboratory, Yale-New Haven Hospital since 1967.[166]

15

OPTIMAL WRIGHT'S STAIN

The optimal Wright's staining reaction is pink upon gross observation. The area between the cells should be free of artefacts. The rbcs should be pink, not reddish-orange or blue-green. The polymorphonuclear leukocyte is the best leukocyte to examine for optimal staining results because of the contrast between acidophilic and basophilic components in this cell. The nucleus of the polymorphonuclear leukocyte is a deep blue-purple and the cytoplasm granules a lilac or violet pink. With Romanowsky dyes, acidic groupings of nucleic acids and proteins of cell nuclei and immature or reactive cytoplasm take up the basic dye, methylene blue, while basic groupings of hemoglobin molecules result in affinity for acidic dyes and staining by eosin.[44]

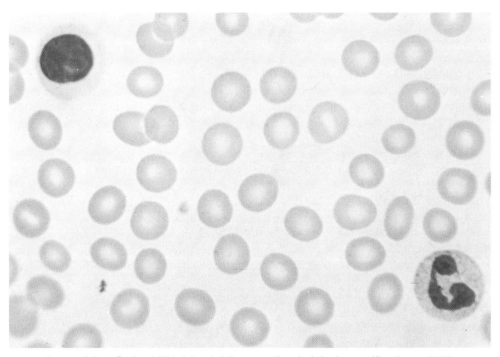

Figure 4.1.   Optimal Wright's staining reaction (original magnification ×600).

TOO ACIDIC WRIGHT'S STAIN

If the Wright's staining reaction is too acidic or too red, the nuclear chromatin of the leukocytes and other structures which usually take the basophilic stain are pale blue rather than a bright, vivid blue and the erythrocytes stain a bright red-orange. Eosinophilic granules display a brilliant red-orange staining reaction.[77,164,185,186]

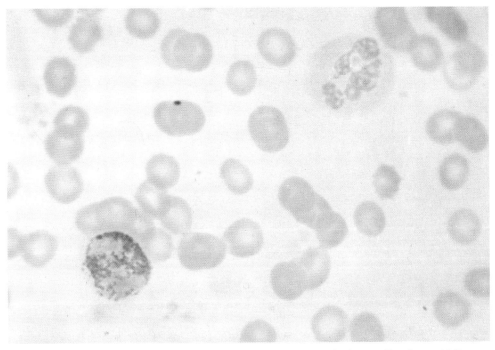

Figure 4.2.   Too acidic Wright's staining reaction (original magnification ×600).

A too acidic Wright's stain may be due to

1. Insufficient staining time.
2. Prolonged buffering or washing.
3. Too acidic stain, buffer, or water which may be due to exposure of stain or buffer to acid fumes or it may be old stain in which the methyl alcohol has slowly oxidized to formic acid.

Remedies

1. Prolong the staining time.
2. Check the pH of stain and buffer and correct with alkali if necessary.
3. Shorten buffering time[77,164,185,186]

TOO ALKALINE WRIGHT'S STAIN

If Wright's stain is too alkaline or too blue, the nuclear chromatin of the leukocytes stains a deep blue-purple and the cytoplasm of lymphocytes becomes gray or lavender so there is difficulty in distinguishing mononuclear cells. The red cells are stained a blue-green which makes the evaluation of polychromasia in these cells impossible. Eosinophil granules become deep gray or blue and the granules of the neutrophil are intensely overstained and may appear larger than normal thereby mimicking "toxic granulation" seen in leukemoid reactions.[31]

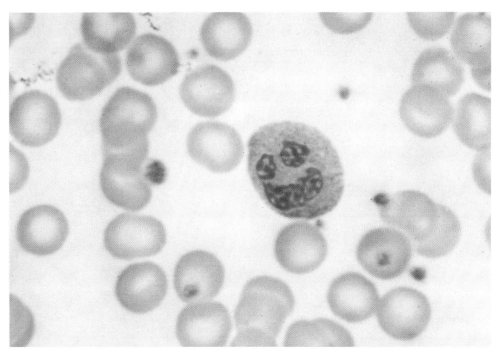

Figure 4.3.   Too alkaline Wright's staining reaction (original magnification ×600).

A too alkaline Wright's stain may be due to:

1. Thick blood smears.
2. Prolonged staining.
3. Insufficient washing.
4. Too alkaline pH of stain, buffer, or water.
5. New stain solution which has not stood for 2–3 weeks may be too basic.

Remedies

1. Check pH of stain, buffer, and water.
2. Shorten staining time.
3. Prolong buffering time.
4. Check the incubation time of the stain.[31,183,185,186]

Table 4.1
Relative and Absolute Values for Leukocyte Counts in Normal Adults per mm^3 Blood[185]

Type of Cell	Relative Value	Absolute Value
	%	number/mm^3
Metamyelocyte	0–1	0–100
Band neutrophil	0–6	0–600
Segmented neutrophil	54–62	2700–6200
Eosinophil	1–3	50–300
Basophil	0–0.75	0–75
Lymphocyte	25–33	1250–3300
Monocyte	3–7	150–700

Normal Adult Total Leukocyte Count/mm^3: 5,000–10,000/mm^3[185]

To derive absolute value range for each type of leukocyte: take the low relative value (%) of the low normal total leukocyte count/mm^3 (5,000) and the high relative value of the high normal total leukocyte count/mm^3.

For example, Eosinophil: 1–3% normal relative value range
5,000–10,000/mm^3 normal total leukocyte count range.

Low absolute eosinophil value:

$5,000 \times 0.01 = 50.00$

High absolute eosinophil value:

$10,000 \times 0.03 = 300.000$

Absolute range for eosinophils:

$50–300/mm^3$

Manual Peripheral Blood Differential Procedure[166]

The first evaluation that must be made by the technologist when performing a peripheral blood differential examination is:

1. **Low Power (10 × Objective and 10 × Ocular) Examination**
   a. *To determine staining characteristics:* see optimal Wright's stain, p. 16.
   b. *To determine distribution of cells*
      1. *Check for isolated large platelet clumps* on fingerstick smears which might result in erroneous low machine counts and low differential platelet estimates by technologist.
      2. *Check for the presence of rouleaux formation of the erythrocytes.*
      3. *Check for the artefactual leukocyte clumping* which results from inadequate mixing of blood sample immediately after collection causing minute fibrin to form to which the leukocytes adhere giving an inaccurate distribution of cell types for the differential examination.
   c. *To select the best area for detailed morphological evaluation*
      1. Edges of erythrocytes not quite touching each other.
      2. Devoid of broken areas.
      3. No flattening or distortion of erythrocytes causing a spurious macrocytosis usually seen at the extreme periphery of the blood smear.
2. **The 50X Oil Immersion Objective and 10X Ocular Examination**
   a. *To determine smear estimate of total leukocyte count/mm³:* Count the number of *both intact and disrupted wbcs* in each of 10 microscopic fields in different areas of the slide where the erythrocytes *slightly* overlap under 50X oil immersion objective. Divide the total number by 10 to establish the mean number of wbcs/field and multiply this mean by 3,000 to get the estimated wbc count/mm³. *Do not truncate the mean*, e.g., if the mean is 5.7 do not truncate to 6 but leave the figure exact to one place past the decimal point for greater accuracy. If the quantitative leukocyte count/mm³ is less than 25,000, the estimated smear count should be within 1,500 cells of this figure. This is less reliable above 25,000 cells/mm³.
3. **The 50X Oil Immersion Objective or 100X Oil Immersion Objective and 10X Ocular Examination**
   Note: The 50X oil immersion objective is recommended for the performance of the 100-cell differential for experienced morphologists because it enhances speed without sacrificing accuracy especially on low white blood cell counts (below 4,000/mm³).
   Note: I would recommend the 100X oil immersion objective for beginning morphologists until they become familiar with the various cell types.
   a. *Adoption of scanning pattern:* a consistent pattern to the direction of traversing microscopic fields is essential to avoid counting the same cell twice.
      1. Scan 10 microscopic fields in a horizontal line proceeding from left to right.
      2. Move slide to next lower field by moving the bottom-most cell in the 10th field of the first horizontal line to just beyond the top of the next lower field. For example,

---

The disrupted leukocytes must be counted in your total leukocyte count/mm³ estimate as intact and disrupted cells would both be counted by the automatic counter since these machines cannot make this distinction. It is highly probable that disrupted wbcs may be incurred in the preparation of the peripheral blood smear and yet represent intact wbcs in the venous sample counted by machine.

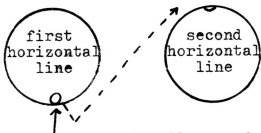

move bottommost cell upward with vertical slide
adjustment knob

3. Proceed from right to left in a horizontal line, repeating this procedure until 100 leukocytes have been counted. For example,

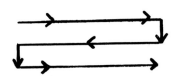

SCANNING PATTERN

ILLUSTRATION

b. A 100-cell differential count of leukocytes is performed using a multiple unit cell tabulator, the above scanning pattern, and either 50X or 100X oil immersion objectives and 10X ocular lenses. Do not include cells other than leukocytes in your 100-cell differential such as nucleated red blood cells or nucleated mega-karyocytic cells, etc.

c. The following leukocytes are included in the 100-cell differential count:
    1. Abnormal precursor.
    2. Blast.
    3. Promyelocyte.
    4. Neutrophilic myelocyte.
    5. Neutrophilic metamyelocyte.
    6. Neutrophilic band.
    7. Neutrophilic segmented form.
    8. Neutrophilic hypersegmented form.
    9. Neutrophilic hypersegmented macrocytic form.
    10. Eosinophilic myelocyte.
    11. Eosinophilic metamyelocyte.
    12. Eosinophilic band.
    13. Eosinophilic segmented form (eosinophil).
    14. Basophilic myelocyte.
    15. Basophilic metamyelocyte.
    16. Basophilic band.
    17. Basophilic segmented form (basophil).
    18. Immature lymphocyte (prolymphocyte).
    19. Mature lymphocyte.
    20. Atypical lymphocyte.
    21. Immature monocyte (promonocyte).
    22. Mature monocyte.
    23. Atypical monocyte.
    24. Proplasma cell.
    25. Mature plasma cell.

d. Any leukocyte containing an abnormal inclusion within its cytoplasm shall be included within the 100-cell differential count, but, in addition, a separate count of those cells with inclusions shall be made on a piece of paper and a written notation of the percentage of cells and type of inclusion shall be made on the patient's requisition slip.

For example, polymorphonuclear leukocytes containing Döhle bodies:

1. Punch polymorphonuclear leukocytes with Döhle bodies into the polymorphonuclear leukocyte column of the multiple unit tabulator.
2. Keep separate numerical count of these cells on piece of paper: ||| ||| |||
3. Record on bottom of patient's requisition slip: 20% polymorphonuclear leukocytes exhibit Döhle bodies.

This procedure should be followed for leukocytes containing the following inclusions:

    Döhle bodies.
    Auer rods.
    Pelger-Huet nuclei.
    May-Hegglin anomaly.
    Alder-Reilly inclusions.
    Chediak-Higashi inclusions.
    toxic granulation.

e. The following cells are counted and reported as the number of cells/100 wbcs on the differential smear, but they are not included in the 100-cell differential count because they are not leukocytes:

    Nucleated erythrocytes.
    Megakaryocytic series: megakaryoblast, promegakaryocyte, megakaryocyte.
    Endothelial cells.
    Epithelial cells.
    Smudged undifferentiated cells.
    Unidentifiable polynuclear cell.
    Unidentifiable mononuclear cell.

For example, if you see 4 nucleated rbcs as you count 100 leukocytes, record them on a separate piece of paper ||| but do *not* punch them into the multiple unit cell tabulator. You have actually counted 104 cells in total: 100 leukocytes and 4 nucleated red blood cells. Record the number of nucleated red blood cells at the bottom of the patient's requisition slip separately.

f. When 6 or more nucleated red blood cells or nonleukocyte nucleated cells (*e.g.*, megakaryoblasts) are seen per 100 leukocytes on a peripheral blood smear, the total leukocyte count/mm^3 must be corrected and reported. The formula to use for correction is:

$$\frac{\text{Leukocyte count/mm}^3 \times 100}{100 + \text{number of nucleated red blood cells}} = \text{corrected wbc/mm}^3$$

4. **The 100X Oil Immersion Objective and 10X Ocular Examination**

a. *The performance of erythrocyte morphology evaluation:* Scan 10 microscopic fields in different areas of the slide with evenly dispersed red blood cells for the erythrocyte morphology evaluation using the 100X oil immersion objective *ONLY*. Please use the following criteria. They are *not absolute* but serve as a *helpful guideline* for evaluating slight, moderate, or marked degrees of hypochromia, anisocytosis, poikilocytosis, and polychromasia of red blood cells based on fields containing 97–162 cells. This procedure will provide a qualitative estimation of a patient's red blood cell morphology.

1. *Hypochromia*: when an individual rbc contains a central pale area which is greater than one-third the diameter of the cell, it is termed a hypochromic cell. Count the hypochromic cells in 10 microscopic fields of evenly dispersed red blood cells. Divide the total of these fields by 10 to establish the mean figure. Match this mean figure to the following guidelines for slight, moderate, and marked degrees of hypochromia or normal, and record on patient's requisition slip.

Table 4.2
Mean Ranges for Hypochromic Red Blood Cells/10 Fields

Normochromia	Slight Hypochromia	Moderate Hypochromia	Marked Hypochromia
0–5	6–15	16–30	↑30

Note: Hyperchromia is *not* reported but is noted in order to correlate with the observation of spherocytes. This term applies to red blood cells which appear deeper in color than the normal red blood cells indicating a higher hemoglobin content to the cell than the volume of the cell should contain.

2. *Anisocytosis: (Erythrocyte size)*

    Definition: Normocyte 6–8 μ

                 Macrocyte 9–↑ μ

                 Microcyte 3–5 μ

    Count the macrocytic and/or microcytic red blood cells *separately* in 10 microscopic fields of evenly dispersed rbcs. Divide the total of these fields by 10 to establish the mean figure. Match this mean figure to the following guidelines for slight, moderate, or marked degrees of anisocytosis or normal, and record on patient's requisition slip.

Table 4.3
Mean Ranges for Anisocytosis/10 Fields of Red Blood Cells

Normal	Slight Anisocytosis	Moderate Anisocytosis	Marked Anisocytosis
0–5	6–15	15–30	↑30

If there is only an increase in macrocytic rbcs, then the mean for macrocytosis and total anisocytosis will be the same and both would be reported as slight, for example, if the mean figure was 8. This would also be true if only an increase in microcytic rbcs was noted on the peripheral blood smear. If both macrocytic and microcytic rbcs exceed the normal mean range, then a mean for each will be established, for example: mean for macrocytosis is 10 and mean for microcytosis is 12 so you would report slight macrocytosis and slight microcytosis on the patient's requisition slip and record the total anisocytosis as moderate since the total of the two means would be 22. Once the peripheral blood differential evaluation for hypochromia and anisocytosis is determined using the numerical guidelines in Tables 4.2 and 4.3, and a Coulter S profile on a patient is performed, then Tables 4.4 and 4.5, which tell the appropriate correlation between the smear evaluation for hypochromia and anisocytosis and the Coulter S parameters mean corpuscular volume (MCV) and mean corpuscular hemoglobin concentration (MCHC), respectively, can be referred to. This serves as a crude method of quality control.

Table 4.4
Red Blood Cell Hypochromia Correlation with Coulter S Parameter MCHC

Smear Evaluation	MCHC Coulter S
Normochromia	31.5–36
Hypochromia	
Slight	30.0–31.5
Moderate	29.0–30.5
Marked	↓29

Note: Recheck any MCHC over 36% for hemolysis, cold agglutinins, or insufficient blood in relation to EDTA.

Table 4.5
Red Blood Cell Anisocytosis Correlation with Coulter S Parameter MCV

Smear Evaluation	MCV Coulter S
Marked microcytosis	↓65
Moderate microcytosis	66–75
Slight microcytosis	
Male	76–79
Female	76–80
Normal	
Male	80–94
Female	81–100
Slight macrocytosis	
Male	95–108
Female	101–108
Moderate macrocytosis	109–120
Marked macrocytosis	↑120

3. *Poikilocytosis:* (*Erythrocyte shape*)
   If only one abnormal shape is noted on a smear and the mean figure falls in the "slight" range, then report that abnormal shape as slight and the total poikilocytosis evaluation would also be slight. For example, slight target cells, slight poikilocytosis. If, however, there are several abnormal red blood cell shapes on one peripheral blood smear, establish the mean for each abnormal shape and report as such on the patient's requisition slip. Total all these means to derive the total poikilocytosis for this patient, *e.g.*,

   Target cell mean   3
   Spherocyte mean   3
   Ovalocyte mean   4
   Burr cell mean   6

   Total mean   16
   Report total poikilocytosis as marked!

Please refer to pages 26–28 for schematic diagrams of each type of poikilocyte and the diseases in which they are most commonly seen in the peripheral blood.

Note: Each abnormal red blood cell shape must be evaluated *SEPARATELY*! Count the number of a particular abnormal red blood cell shape in 10 microscopic fields. Divide the total number by 10 to derive the mean figure for that particular abnormal shape. Match this mean figure to the following guidelines for evaluating red blood cell poikilocytosis.

Table 4.6.
Mean Ranges for Poikilocytosis of Red Blood Cells/10 Fields

Abnormal Shape	Normal	Slight	Moderate	Marked
Spherocyte	0	1–5	6–15	↑15
Acanthocyte	0	1–5	6–15	↑15
Sickle cell	0	1–5	6–15	↑15
Rouleaux forms	0	1–5	6–15	↑15
Envelope forms	0–1	2–5	6–15	↑15
Tear drop forms	0–1	2–5	6–15	↑15
Bizarre forms	0–1	2–5	6–15	↑15
Tailed rbc forms	0–1	2–5	6–15	↑15
Target cells	0–1	2–5	6–15	↑15
Schistocytes	0–1	2–5	6–15	↑15
Ovalocytes	0–1	2–5	6–15	↑15
Elliptocytes	0–1	2–5	6–15	↑15
Burr cells	0–1	2–5	6–15	↑15
Stomatocytes	0–1	2–5	6–15	↑15
Blister cells	0–1	2–5	6–15	↑15

4. *Polychromasia: (Rbc Immaturity)*

    Count the polychromatophilic (gray-blue) red blood cells in 10 microscopic fields containing evenly dispersed red blood cells. Divide the total of these fields by 10 to establish the mean figure. Match this mean figure to the following guidelines for slight, moderate, or marked polychromatophilia or normal, and record on the patient's requisition slip.

ERYTHROCYTE POIKILOCYTOSIS

NORMOCHROMIC, NORMOCYTIC RBC

TARGET CELL (LEPTOCYTE):

Liver disease
Artefact
Thalassemia major
Thalassemia minor
Sickle cell anemia
C-C disease
Sickle-thalassemia
S-C disease
A-C and A-S traits
Post-splenectomy
Moderate to severe iron
deficiency

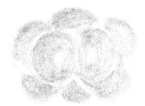

AGGLUTINATION:

Cold agglutinins
Autoimmune hemolytic anemia
Macroglobulinemia (Waldenstrom's)
Increased gamma globulins

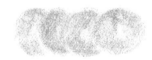

ROULEAUX FORMATION:

Multiple myeloma
Macroglobulinemia (Waldenstrom's)
Increased gamma globulins

NORMOCHROMIC OVALOCYTE:

Hereditary ovalocytosis
Sickle cell anemia
Thalassemia major

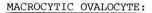

HYPOCHROMIC OVALOCYTE:

Moderate to severe iron
deficiency

MACROCYTIC OVALOCYTE:

Megaloblastic anemias:
B_{12} deficiency and
Folate deficiency

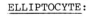

ELLIPTOCYTE:

Hereditary elliptocytosis
Megaloblastic anemias
Myelofibrosis
Thalassemia major
Artefact
Mechanical trauma

Figure 4.4.   *A to C,* erythrocyte poikilocytosis.

ERYTHROCYTE POIKILOCYTOSIS

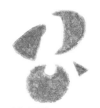

BLISTER CELL:

Microangiopathic hemolytic
anemia

SCHISTOCYTES:
(FRAGMENTED RBCS)

Microangiopathic
hemolytic anemia
(Waring blender
 syndrome)
Hypersplenism
Myeloid metaplasia
Megaloblastic anemia
Thalassemia major
Acute Leukemia (post
therapy)
Post severe burns
Hemolytic anemias
Enzyme deficiencies

TAILED RBC:

Megaloblastic anemias:
B_{12} deficiency and
Folate deficiency
Myeloid metaplasia
Moderate to severe
iron deficiency

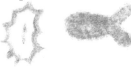

TEAR DROP FORM (DACRYOCYTE):

Myeloid metaplasia
Hypersplenism
Thalassemia major and minor
Acquired hemolytic anemias
Megaloblastic anemias

BIZARRE RBC FORMS:

Used for rbc forms that
do not fit into any
specified rbc category
for poikilocytosis

ANULOCYTE: (severely hypochromic
                        cell)

Moderate to severe iron deficiency
Thalassemia major and minor
(does not represent a poikilocyte,
 but included here so term "anulocyte"
 would not be confused with descriptive terms of known poikilocytes)

ACHROMOCYTE (SEMI-LUNAR
                        BODY)

Occasionally seen on
peripheral blood smears.
Not associated with any
specific disease state.
Disintegrating rbc which
assumes a crescent shape
not to be confused with
a sickle cell. Achromo-
cytes stain faintly whereas sickle cells are very
well-stained with Wright's
stain

Figure 4.4B.

ERYTHROCYTE POIKILOCYTOSIS

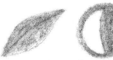

ENVELOPE FORMS:

Hgb C-C disease
S-C disease
C-Thalassemia
Thalassemia major
Liver disease
Sickle-Thalassemia
A-C trait

STOMATOCYTES:

Hereditary stomatocytosis
Artefact
Acute leukemia, treated
occasionally
Alcoholics with liver
disease occasionally
Severe infection rarely

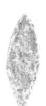 

OAT   FILAMENTOUS
CELL   FORM
FORM
        OF
SICKLE CELLS (DREPANOCYTES):

Sickle cell anemia
S-C disease
Sickle-Thalassemia

SPHEROCYTES:

Hereditary spherocytosis
ABO incompatibility
Autoimmune hemolytic
anemia
Microangiopathic hemolytic
anemia
Hypersplenism
Myeloid metaplasia
Post-splenectomy
Post-severe burns
Hemoglobinopathies
Malaria
Artefact - thin area of
smear
Older population of trans-
fused cells
Liver disease

BURR CELLS (KERATOCYTES):

Hemolytic anemias:
Microangiopathic hemolytic anemia
Moderate to severe iron deficiency
Megaloblastic anemias
Thalassemia major and minor
Myeloid metaplasia
Hypersplenism

ACANTHOCYTES:

Abetalipoproteinemia
Hemolytic anemias:
Microangiopathic hemo-
lytic anemia
Autoimmune hemolytic
anemia
Sideroblastic anemia
Thalassemia major
Liver disease
Severe burns
Post splenectomy
Renal disease
Enzyme deficiencies

Figure 4.4C.

Table 4.7
Mean Ranges for Polychromasia of Red Blood Cells/10 Fields and
Corresponding Reticulocyte Values

Normal	Slight	Moderate	Marked
0–1.5	1.6–2.5	2.6–3.5	↑ 3.6
0–2%	2–4%	4–6%	↑ 6%
	Reticulocyte Values		

The above reticulocyte percentages were obtained by counting the number of reticulocytes seen per 1,000 red blood cells on new methylene blue-stained smears and converting to per cent.

5. *Erythrocyte Inclusions*

Count the red blood cells containing one particular type of inclusion in each of 10 microscopic fields of evenly dispersed red blood cells. Divide the total of these fields by 10 to establish the mean figure. Match this mean figure to the following guidelines for slight, moderate, marked, or normal and record on patient's requisition slip. Please refer to pages 30–31 for photographs of these red blood cell inclusions.

Note: Repeat this above procedure for *each* type of red blood cell inclusion on the smear.

Table 4.8
Mean Ranges for Erythrocyte Inclusions/10 Fields

Type of Inclusion	Normal	Slight	Moderate	Marked
Howell-Jolly body Pappenheimer body Cabot ring Basophilic stippling	None	1–2	3–5	↑ 6

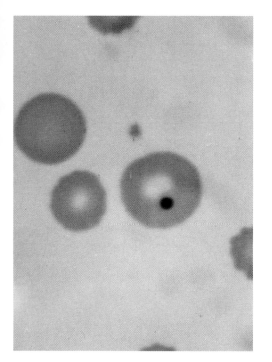
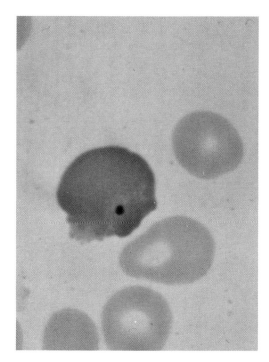

Figure 4.5.   Howell-Jolly body (original magnification ×1500).

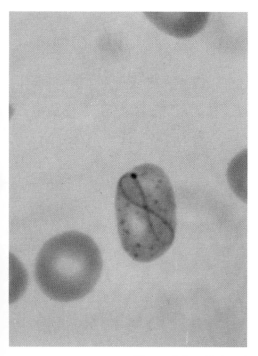
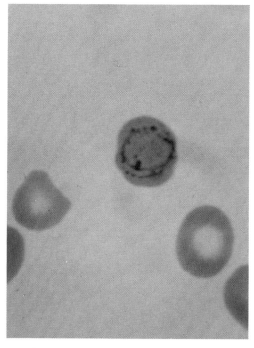

Figure 4.6.   Cabot ring (original magnification ×1500).

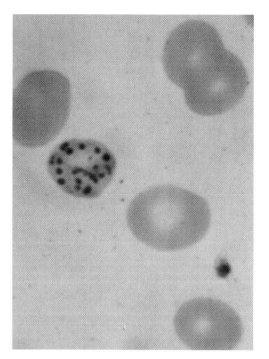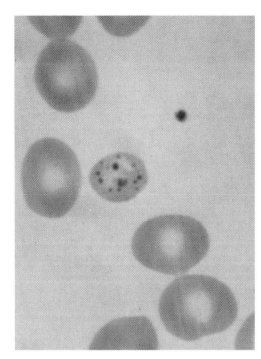

Figure 4.7. Basophilic stippling (original magnification ×1500). Left, coarse. *Right*, fine.

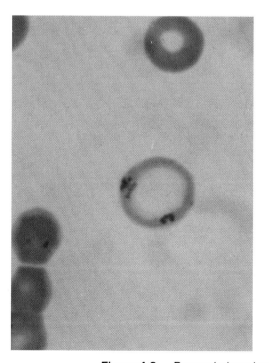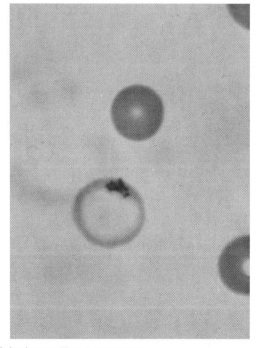

Figure 4.8. Pappenheimer bodies (original magnification ×1500).

b. *To determine smear estimate of the total platelet count/mm^3:*
Count the number of platelets in each of 10 microscopic fields in different areas of the slide where the red blood cells are evenly dispersed. Avoid fields in which red blood cells strongly overlap as this will falsely increase the platelet estimate. Watch for platelets that may be superimposed on erythrocytes and include in your count. Divide the total number of platelets by 10 to establish the mean figure and multiply this mean by 13,000 to get the estimated platelet count/mm^3. Do not truncate the mean figure, *e.g.*, if the mean is 8.6, do not truncate to 9 but leave the figure exactly one place past the decimal point for greater accuracy.

Note: If small to moderately sized clumps of platelets are seen in a consistent pattern throughout the smear and the individual platelets are easily discernible, attempt a smear estimate of platelets and compare to a platelet count performed by phase microscopy. If the smear estimate and the phase platelet count do not check within the allowable error, report only the smear estimate of platelets since an accurate count/mm^3 is impossible due to clumping.

Table 4.9
Mean Ranges for Smear Estimates of Platelets/10 Fields with Estimates of Platelet Counts/mm^3 and Methods of Reporting

Mean Ranges for Smear Estimates of Platelets/10 Fields	Estimated Platelet Count/mm^3	Report as
0–3	0–50,000	Markedly reduced
4–7	50,000–100,000	Moderately reduced
8–11	100,000–150,000	Slightly reduced
12–27	150,000–350,000	Adequate or normal
↑ 28	↑ 350,000	Numerous

If the quantitative platelet count/mm^3 is less than 300,000 and greater than 75,000/mm^3, then the estimated smear count should be within 26,000/mm^3 or a two platelet mean of this figure. If the platelet count is less than 75,000/mm^3, then the estimated smear count should be within 13,000/mm^3 or a one-platelet mean of the quantitative platelet count/mm^3. If the quantitative platelet count is greater than 300,000/mm^3, then the smear estimate should be within 52,000 or a four-platelet mean of this figure.

Automated Differential Leukocyte Counting Machines

The automated differential leukocyte counting machines that have been developed to date employ either a flow system which analyzes cell size and biochemical parameters for cellular identification or a pattern recognition system which identifies cells on fixed, stained blood films prepared by the traditional "wedge" technique or by a "spinner" method.[139, 140]

The flow systems afford a rapid analysis of large numbers of cells (*e.g.*, 10,000–12,000 cells/min in each channel), thereby increasing the accuracy of the count over the manual differential counts of 100 or more cells. The flow systems also enhance the detection of cells usually present in small numbers. Cell size is determined by measurement of light scattering or conductivity. Cells such as leukocytes are also characterized by measurement of light absorption of either unstained or stained cells, or fluorescence of cellular constituents after staining with fluorescent dyes. Erythrocyte interference is avoided by hemolysis with lytic agents and platelets do not interfere because of their small size.[184]

The Technicon H6000 is a flow system which measures nine parameters: 1) white blood cell count; 2) white blood cell differential count: a) neutrophils, b) lymphocytes, c) monocytes, d) eosinophils, e) basophils, f) LUC (large unidentified cells), g) HPX (cells with high peroxidase activity); 3) hematocrit; 4) hemoglobin; 5) red blood cell count; 6) MCV (mean corpuscular volume); 7) MCH (mean corpuscular hemoglobin); 8) MCHC (mean corpuscular hemoglobin concentration); and 9) platelet count.

The Technicon H6000 aspirates $300/\mu l$ of EDTA-anticoagulated whole blood at room temperature at the rate of 60 samples per hour. To ensure a homogeneous sample, each specimen is stirred by a mixing paddle immediately before it is aspirated. The aspirated sample is then diluted, divided into three streams—one for each of three analytical manifolds. *Note:* This system may be equipped with the optional Technicon Autoslide System. In that case, 550 μl of whole blood is aspirated, and 250 μl of this sample is used to prepare a stained smear on mylar film which is mounted on a glass slide. The flow of fluids (except the blood specimen) through this system is controlled by four pneumatically actuated pinch valves. Depending upon the operational mode, the pinch valves rotate water, reagents, and wash solutions through the system. The rbc/plt/hgb manifold contains two channels: a hgb channel and a rbc/plt channel. Upon entering the rbc/plt/hgb manifold, the sample is diluted and resampled to each of these two channels. In the hgb channel, the hgb diluent reagent converts the blood sample's hemoglobin to cyanmethemoglobin. The resulting solution flows to the hemoglobin colorimeter and is read. The hgb colorimeter has a sample channel and a reference channel. The sample channel measures the absorbance (A) of the hgb analytical stream as it passes through a flow cell. Light transmitted through the flow cell at a wavelength of 550 nm is converted to an electrical signal by a photomultiplier tube (PMT). The reference channel is optically identical to the sample channel (except that there is no flow cell) and is used to compensate for any variation in the output of the optics lamp. Electrical outputs from the sample and reference phototubes are applied to hgb signal processing circuits. In the rbc/plt channel, the sample is diluted and then routed to rbc/plt optics where light scattering characteristics of the sample are measured. Particles (cells) in the sample scatter light in direct proportion to their size. The rbc/plt Optics Assembly contains two detection channels. In one channel, the light-scattering characteristics of the sample are measured by a photodiode. This channel is used to enumerate red blood cells. The hematocrit is determined by integrating the light-scattering signals for the detected red cell population, then multiplying the result by a suitable calibration constant. In the second channel, the light-scattering characteristics of the sample are measured by a PMT. The greater sensitivity provided by the PMT allows quantitative detection of the lower levels of light that are scattered by the smaller-sized platelets. The electrical outputs from the photodiode and the PMT are applied to the rbc/plt signal processing circuits.

In the alkaline peroxidase manifold, the enzymes within the white blood cells are stained cytochemically. The degree to which a particular cell is stained and the light scattering characteristics of the cell are the criteria for classifying specific cell types. The total white blood cell count, the neutrophil percent of white blood cells, the monocyte percent of white blood cells, the lymphocyte percent of white blood cells, the eosinophil percent of white blood cells, LUC percent of white blood cells, and cells with HPX percent of white blood cells are measured in the alkaline peroxidase manifold.

The enzyme peroxidase is present and active in several leukocyte cell types. In the presence of hydrogen peroxide and an appropriate electron receptor chromogen, peroxidase develops a darkly colored precipitate. Eosinophils and neutrophils contain peroxidases that are still active at low pH with eosinophils retaining peroxidase activity at pH 2 (low peroxidase cells). However, there is sufficient difference in staining intensity of neutrophils and eosinophils at higher values to permit electro-optical separation of two cell types using only the neutrophil manifold. With the use of electronic thresholds to separate cell types, the original, low pH peroxidase manifold became unnecessary. The low amounts of peroxidase in monocytes define them as a cell population with large scatter signals and absorption signals that extend from unstained cells up to and partially overlapping weakly stained neutrophils. Improvement in fixation technique allows more complete separation of monocytes signals in the peroxidase channel from LUC and neutrophils. The mean monocyte absorption signal is about one-third that of neutrophils. A separate monocyte channel is no longer necessary. The alkaline peroxidase channel counts three populations of stained cells (neutrophils, monocytes, and eosinophils), two populations of unstained cells (lymphocytes and LUC) with great precision.

In the basophil manifold, red blood cells are lysed, and basophils are preferentially stained with Alcian blue. The analytical stream from this manifold is applied to the basophil optics. The electro-optical detection system consists of four optical assemblies that are axially positioned about a common tungsten-halogen light source (optics lamp). The Basophil Optics Assembly contains two scatter channels. One channel measures light-scattering characteristics of the sample at "red" wavelengths, while the other channel measures light-scattering at "green" (red to green) wavelengths. Outputs from "red" and "green" scatter photodiodes are applied to basophil signal-processing circuits. Basophilic granules are strongly anionic due to their heparin content. Based on this fact, acridine orange, neutral red, toluidine blue, and Alcian blue have been suggested as possible stains for basophils. Alcian blue is the stain of choice for the Technicon H6000 system because it produces greater contrast and its absorption spectrum better matches the optical parameters of the system. Implicit in the use of Alcian blue dye is close pH control (2.2) since at any other pH there would be a tendency for all nuclei to stain. In addition, at the low pH the hemoglobin in the sample converts to acid hematin. The molar extinction of acid hematin is only 7% that of hemoglobin resulting in increased method sensitivity due to decreased background absorbance of the suspending fluid.

The above information on the Technicon H6000 system was taken from the Technicon Product Labeling Manual for the H6000 System—Technical Publication No. UA80-443A00.

Pattern recognition or digital image processing systems utilize blood films prepared on glass slides by the traditional "wedge" technique or by a "spinner" method. The slide is then placed on the microscope stage which is driven by a motor. A computer controls the movement scanning the slide, stopping it whenever leukocytes are in the field of vision. The optical images, *e.g.*, nuclear size, shape, and color and cytoplasmic size and color, are recorded by a television camera, analyzed by the computer, and then converted to digital form.[187] These characteristics are then compared with a memory bank of such characteristics for the different cell types. If the pattern "fits" that of a normal cell type it is identified as such, otherwise, it is classified as an unknown. The coordinates of the unknown cells can be kept by some instruments and can be relocated at the end of the count so the technologist can classify them by visual identification.

The Coulter Diff 3 (formerly the Cell Scan-Glopr), which was originally developed by the Perkin-Elmer Corporation, is such a pattern recognition instrument which has the potential of closely duplicating human interpretation of the normal blood film. It utilizes a "spinner"-prepared, stained blood film to perform a differential leukocyte count, evaluate red blood cell morphology, and estimate the number of platelets (high, normal, or low). The computer on the Coulter Diff 3 is programmed to classify 11 cell types: 1) band neutrophil, 2) segmented neutrophil, 3) lymphocyte, 4) monocyte, 5) eosinophil, 6) basophil, 7) nucleated red blood cell, 8) atypical lymphocyte, 9) blast cell, 10) immature granulocyte, and 11) "other" unclassified cell.

Geometric Data's Hematrak is a pattern recognition instrument which analyzes either a "wedge" type manually prepared blood film or a "spinner" blood film. It provides automated red blood cell morphology, enumeration of reticulocytes, numeric platelet estimates, leukocyte measurement indices, and Price-Jones red blood cell size distribution. The computer on the Hematrak classifies 10 cell types: 1) segmented neutrophils, 2) band neutrophils, 3) lymphocytes, 4) eosinophils, 5) basophils, 6) monocytes, 7) nucleated red blood cells, 8) atypical lymphocytes, 9) suspect cells, and 10) reticulocytes.

The Abbott ADC 500 is a third pattern recognition instrument used to perform a differential leukocyte count, evaluate red blood cell morphology, and estimate the sufficiency of platelets. The computer is programmed to classify the following cell types: 1) segmented neutrophils, 2) band neutrophils, 3) lymphocytes, 4) monocytes, 5) eosinophils, 6) basophils, 7) atypical lymphocytes, 8) immature granulocytes, 9) blast cells, 10) nucleated red blood cells, and 11) unclassifed cells.

Table 4.10
Comparative Chart of Instruments for Differential Counts

	Technicon H600	Coulter Diff 3	Abbott ADC 500	Geometric Data Hematrak
Principle of operation	Cytochemical and electro-optical technique	Computerized pattern recognition	Computerized pattern recognition	Computerized pattern recognition
Samples/hr	60 Samples/hr Sample batch 40	30–35 samples/hr Sample batch 14	40 samples/hr at 500 cells/sample	30–50 samples/hr Sample batch 1
Slide type	No slide required but autoslide accessory can by purchased to provide slide	Spun slides only	Spun slides only	Wedge or spun
Stain	Cytochemical: alkaline peroxidase alcian blue	Special Wright's stain sold by Coulter Electronics using a system matched to an Ames Hema-Tek stainer	Modified Wright's stain	Wright's stain
Oil Application	Not applicable unless Autoslide purchased	Automatic	Automatic	Manual or automatic
No: wbcs counted	1,000, 10,000	100 (normal mode), 200, 300, 400, 500 also	500, 1,000	50, 100, 200, 400, 800, 1,000 or continuous
Rbc morphology and platelet estimate	No platelet count performed by H6000	Reports percentage: normocytic, microcytic, macrocytic, normochromic, hypochromic, normal shape poikilocyte, platelet sufficiency as normal increased or decreased	Reports normal to 3+: Anisocytosis, Macrocytosis, Microcytosis, Hypochromia, Poikilocytosis, Polychromasia, Normal rbc/100, Platelet sufficiency estimate	Automated rbc morphology, reticulocytes, numeric platelet estimates, leukocyte measurement indices, Price-Jones rbc size distribution
Cell categories	Neutrophils Lymphocytes Monocytes Eosinophils Basophils LUC HPX	Segmented neutrophils Band neutrophils Lymphocytes Monocytes Eosinophils Basophils Atypical lymphocytes Immature granulocytes Blast cells Nucleated rbcs Other	Segmented neutrophils Band neutrophils Lymphocytes Monocytes Eosinophils Basophils Atypical lymphocytes Immature granulocytes Blast cells Nucleated rbcs Unclassified	Segmented neutrophils Band neutrophils Lymphocytes Eosinophils Basophils Monocytes Nucleated rbcs Atypical lymphocytes Suspect cells Reticulocytes

Chapter 5

The Origin and Development of Blood Cells

Human nerve and muscle cells do not retain proliferative capability after embryonic development and therefore cannot regenerate themselves even under normal conditions. However, this is not true of hematopoietic (blood-forming) cells. They immediately retain the capacity for self-renewal following continual destruction as an ongoing physiologic process.[174]

In the embryo, blood cells originate in mesenchymal tissue from the mesoderm. The sites of hematopoiesis vary in a definite sequence in the embryo and the fetus.[174] The first hematopoiesis occurs in extraembryonic parts such as the blood islands in the yolk sac for the first 2–8 weeks which is termed the mesoblastic period. At approximately 2 months' gestation, hematopoiesis becomes a function of the liver primarily and the spleen secondarily (hepatic period) until the fetus is 5 months old when blood formation shifts to the bone marrow (myeloid period) and lymphatic tissue where hematopoiesis continues throughout the remainder of fetal development and for the duration of life after birth. Lymphatic tissue, which is primarily found in the spleen, lymph nodes, tonsils, intestinal tract, and to a lesser extent in the bone marrow, is the site of formation of lymphocytes and plasma cells. Erythrocytes, blood basophils, neutrophils, eosinophils, monocytes, and megakaryocytes are normally formed in the bone marrow.[186]

The formation of blood cells solely in the bone marrow is referred to as medullary hematopoiesis. The formation of blood cells, which are normally produced in the bone marrow, may occur in other organs (liver, spleen, lymph nodes) in pathologic and reactive blood diseases and this is referred to as extramedullary hematopoiesis. Excessive proliferation of lymphocytes, monocytes, plasma cells, and tissue basophils (mast cells) may occur in the bone marrow.

Megaloblastic erythrocytes are the only cells which normally occur in man for a limited period only, namely in the embryo from the second week of pregnancy, when blood formation begins, to the third month of pregnancy. They are formed exclusively in extraembryonic tissues. In the adult they reappear in megaloblastic diseases such as vitamin B_{12} and folate deficiencies and are formed in the bone marrow.[174]

All mammalian cell renewal systems proliferate through cell division. Blood cells, except for the lymphocyte, differentiate to a point where cell division cannot or does not occur. Therefore, for these cells, replacement requiring stem cells involves cellular division (mitosis) coupled with differentiation (maturation).[184]

Recent evidence from studies of erythropoietin-stimulated bone marrow and myeloid colony-forming cells supports the view that the original stem cell is morphologically indistinguishable from the small or medium-sized lymphocytes found in the bone marrow.[38, 104] It is these cells, separated from other marrow cells by glass wool column filters, that can incorporate thymidine into the nucleus, repopulate the marrow, and form spleen colonies in guinea pigs with the development of lines of erythrocytes, granulocytes, and megakaryocytes. Small lymphocytes found in the peripheral blood or lymph nodes, reticulum cells, granulocytic cells, and erythroblastic cells do not possess this capacity.

In addition to the pluripotential stem cell able to reproduce itself or produce any of the marrow cell lines, multipotential stem cells have been recognized in which one type can form megakaryocytes, monocytes, granulocytes, and erythrocytes while another type can produce B-type and T-type lymphocytes. Still another stem cell has been found which can produce either monocytes or granulocytes. "Committed" or specific stem cells which can produce only one type of cell, such as erythrocytes, have also been confirmed.[104]

Morphologically, stem cells of differential potential probably all look alike.[184]

Table 5.1
Nomenclature Outline

Series Prefix	-blast	Pro-cyte	-cyte	Meta-cyte		
Lympho-	Lymphoblast	Prolymphocyte	Lymphocyte			
Mono-	Monoblast	Promonocyte	Monocyte			
Plasma-	Plasmablast	Proplasmacyte	Plasmacyte			
Megakaryo-	Megakaryoblast	Promegakaryocyte	Megakaryocyte	Metamegakaryocyte	Thrombocyte	
Rubri-	Rubriblast	Prorubricyte	Rubricyte	Metarubricyte	Polychromatic erythrocyte	Mature erythrocyte
Myelo-	Myeloblast	Promyelocyte	Eosinophilic myelocyte	Eosinophilic metamyelocyte	Eosinophilic band	Eosinophilic segmented neutrophil
			Neutrophilic myelocyte	Neutrophilic metamyelocyte	Neutrophilic band	Neutrophilic segmented neutrophil
			Basophilic myelocyte	Basophilic metamyelocyte	Basophilic band	Basophilic segmented neutrophil

Chapter 6

The Myelocytic Series

The Neutrophilic Series

Table 6.1
Morphologic Criteria for Neutrophilic Series
Key Differentiating Feature:
Presence or absence of granules in cell with 3:1 or 4:1 N:C ratio and basophilic cytoplasm.

	Myeloblast	Promyelocyte
Cell size	10–20 μm in diameter	10–20 μm in diameter
Nuclear: cytoplasmic ratio (N:C)	*4:1*	*3:1*
Nuclear shape	Round or oval, slight indentation more commonly seen in leukemic states	Round or oval
Nuclear position	Eccentric or central	Eccentric or central
Nuclear color and chromatin	Light red-purple; fine meshwork with no aggregation of material	Light red-purple, fine meshwork, slight aggregation may be seen at nuclear membrane
Nucleoli	1—5	1–5
Color and amount of cytoplasm	*Basophliic* and scanty	*Basophilic* and slightly increased over myeloblast
Cytoplasmic granules	*Absent*	*Present*, fine azurophilic, nonspecific granules

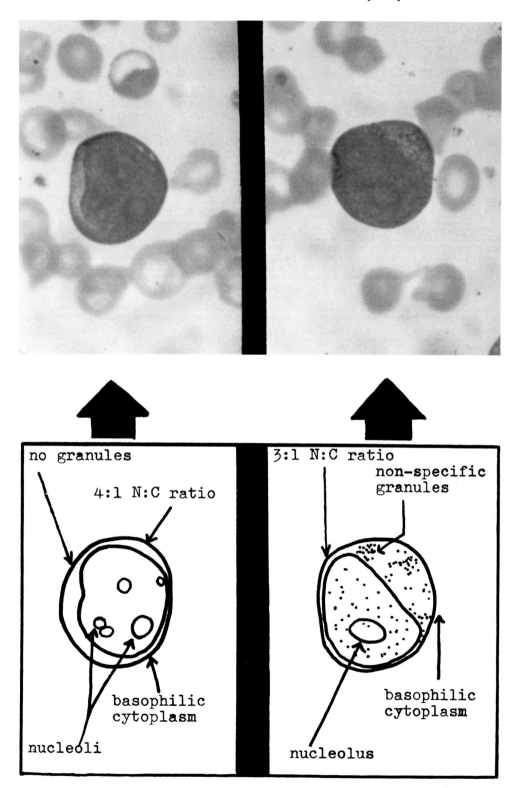

Figure 6.1. *Upper*, myeloblast *versus* promyelocyte. *Lower*, schematic diagram.

Table 6.2
Morphologic Criteria for Neutrophilic Series
Key Differentiating Feature:
The decrease in the nuclear area coupled to a decrease in basophilia of the cytoplasm and the appearance of specific granules.

	Promyelocyte	Myelocyte
Cell size	10–20 μm in diameter	10–18 μm in diameter
Nuclear cytoplasmic ratio (N:C)	*3:1*	*2:1 or 1:1*
Nuclear shape	Round or oval	Oval or slightly indented, occasionally round
Nuclear position	Eccentric or central	Commonly eccentric, may be central
Nuclear color and chromatin	Light red-purple, fine meshwork, slight aggregation may be seen at nuclear membrane in late stages	Red-purple, fine chromatin with slightly aggregated or granular pattern
Nucleoli	1–5	May or may not have nucleolus
Color and amount of cytoplasm	*Basophilic*, slightly increased amount over myeloblast	*Bluish-pink*, moderate
Cytoplasmic granules	Present, fine azurophilic, *nonspecific granules*	Present, azurophilic, *specific granules*, e.g., eosinophilic

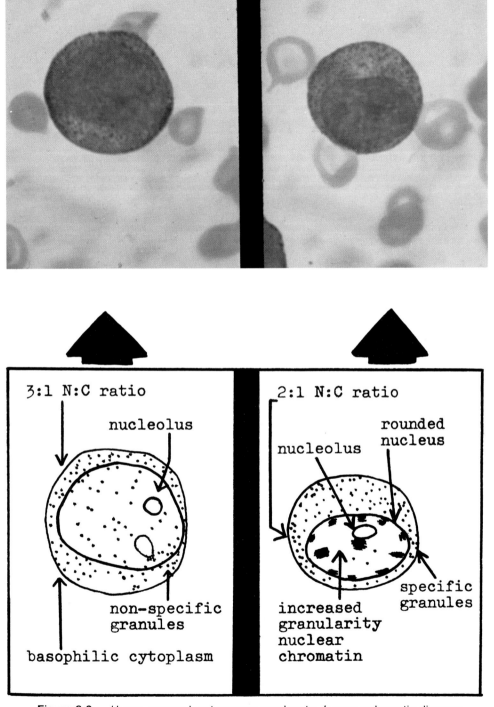

Figure 6.2. *Upper,* promyelocyte *versus* myelocyte. *Lower,* schematic diagram.

Table 6.3
Morphologic Criteria for Neutrophilic Series
Key Differentiating Feature:
Change from fine red-purple chromatin to light blue-purple, distinct basi- and oxychromatin and increased nuclear indentation.

	Myelocyte	Metamyelocyte
Cell size	10–18 μm in diameter	10–18 μm in diameter
Nuclear: cytoplasmic ratio (N:C)	2:1 or 1:1	1:1
Nuclear shape	*Oval*, or slightly indented, *occasionally round*	*Usually indented* (*kidney-shaped*), oval, and rarely round
Nuclear position	Commonly eccentric, may be round	Central or eccentric
Nuclear color and chromatin	*Red-purple fine chromatin* with slightly aggregated or granular pattern	*Light blue-purple with basi- and oxyphilic chromatin easily distinguishable*
Nucleoli	May or may not have nucleoli	None
Color and amount of cytoplasm	Moderate, *bluish-pink*	Moderate, bluish-pink occasionally, *usually clear pink*
Cytoplasmic granules	Present, azurophilic and specific granules, *e.g.*, neutrophilic, eosinophilic	Present, Specific granules, *e.g.*, neutrophilic, eosinophilic

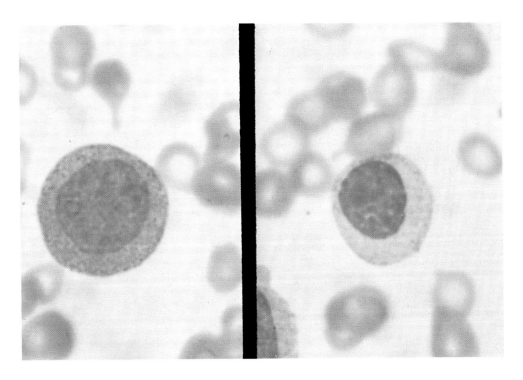

FINE red-purple
nuclear chromatin with
SLIGHT granularity

increased granularity
distinct basi- and
oxy-chromatin seen in
nucleus

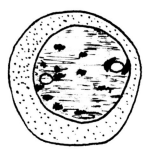

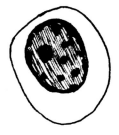

nucleoli

bluish-pink cytoplasm
with specific granules

pink cytoplasm

Figure 6.3.   *Upper*, myelocyte *versus* metamyelocyte. *Lower*, schematic diagram.

Table 6.4
Morphologic Criteria for Neutrophilic Series
Key Differentiating Feature:
Changes from kidney-shaped or wide oval nculeus to narrow elongated band nuclear shape and increased nuclear granularity.

	Metamyelocyte	Band Neutrophil
Cell size	10–18 μm in diameter	10–16 μm in diameter
Nuclear: cytoplasmic ratio (N:C)	1:1	1:1
Nuclear shape	*Usually indented, (kidney-shaped), oval, and rarely round*	*Elongated, narrow band shape of uniform thickness, singular nuclear lobe*
Nuclear position	Central or eccentric	Central or eccentric
Nuclear color and chromatin	*Light blue-purple with basi- and oxyphilic chromatin easily distinguishable*	*Deep blue-purple coarsely granular chromatin*
Nucleoli	None	None
Color and amount of cytoplasm	Moderate, occasionally bluish-pink, usually clear pink	Abundant, pink
Cytoplasmic granules	Specific granules, *e.g.*, neutrophilic, eosinophilic	Specific granules, fine violet-pink

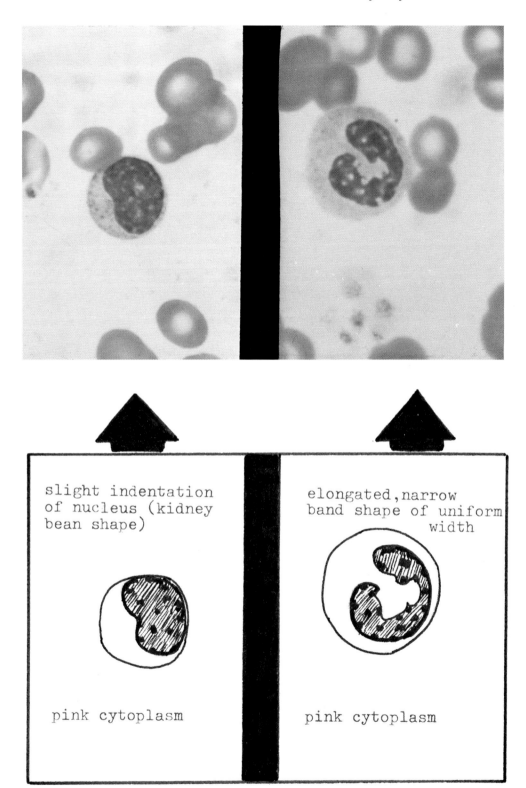

Figure 6.4. *Upper*, metamyelocyte *versus* band neutrophil. *Lower*, schematic diagram.

Table 6.5
Morphologic Criteria for Neutrophilic Series
Key Differentiating Feature:
Changes from elongated, narrow singular nuclear lobe to a multilobed (2–5) nucleus.

	Band Neutrophil	Segmented Neutrophil
Cell size	10–16 μm in diameter	10–16 μm in diameter
Nuclear: cytoplasmic ratio (N:C)	1:1	1:1
Nuclear shape	*Elongated narrow band shape of uniform thickness, singular nuclear lobe*	*2–5 distinct nuclear lobes (0.5 μm filament connecting lobes)*
Nuclear position	Central or eccentric	Central or eccentric
Nuclear color and chromatin	Deep blue-purple coarsely granular chromatin	Deep blue-purple coarsely granular chromatin
Nucleoli	None	None
Color and amount of cytoplasm	Abundant pink	Abundant pink
Cytoplasmic granules	Specific, fine violet-pink	Specific, fine violet-pink

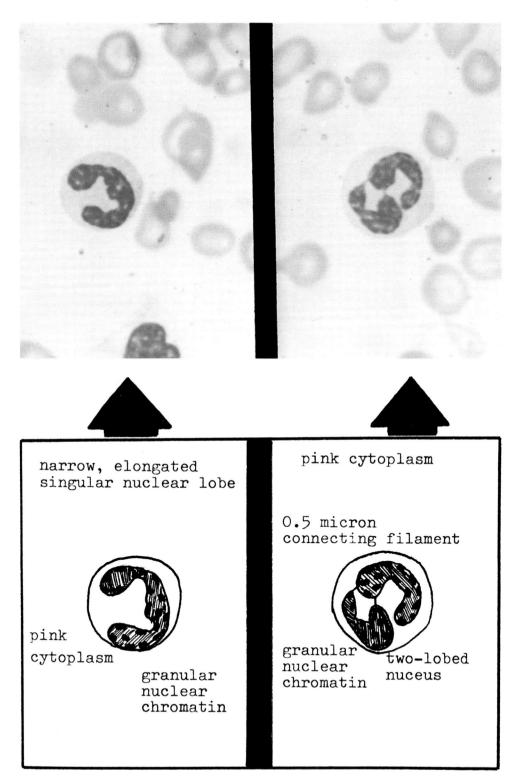

Figure 6.5.   *Upper*, band neutrophil *versus* segmented neutrophil. *Lower*, schematic diagram.

Table 6.6
Morphologic Criteria for Neutrophilic Series
Key Differentiating Feature:
Increase in the number of nuclear lobes from 2–5 to 6 or more.

	Segmented Neutrophil	Hypersegmented Neutrophil
Cell size	10–16 μm in diameter	10–16 or 15–25 μm in diameter
Nuclear cytoplasmic ratio (N:C)	1:1	1:1
Nuclear shape	*2–5 distinct nuclear lobes (0.5 μm filament connecting lobes*	*6–10 or more distinct nuclear lobes (0,.5 μm filament connecting lobes)*
Nuclear position	Central or eccentric	Central or eccentric
Nuclear color and chromatin	Deep blue-purple coarsely granular chromatin	Deep blue-purple coarsely granular chromatin
Nucleoli	None	None
Color and amount of cytoplasm	Abundant pink	Abundant pink
Cytoplasmic granules	Specific, fine violet-pink	Specific, fine violet-pink

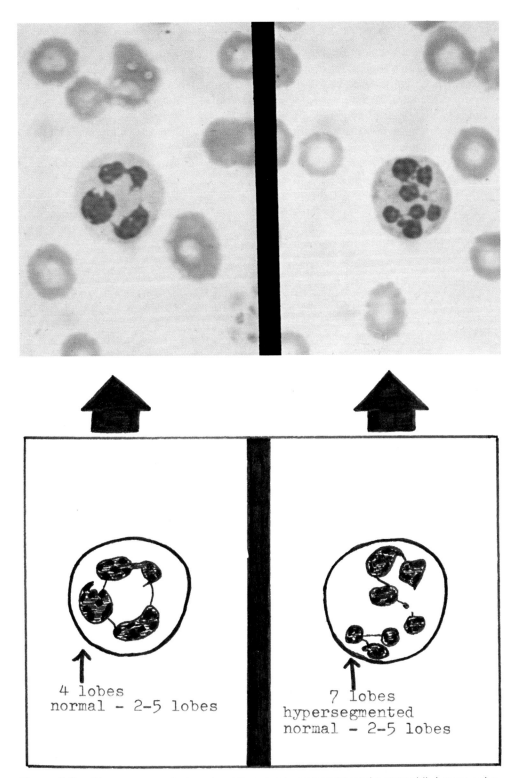

Figure 6.6.   *Upper*, segmented neutrophil *versus* hypersegmented neutrophil. *Lower*, schematic diagram.

NECROBIOSIS OF BLOOD CELLS

The liquefied nucleus of disintegrating cells, even segmented forms, either coalesces to form one large round drop or scatters into several small droplets. When the nucleus liquefies, the viscous, basophilic chromatin frequently separates from the thinly liquid, oxyphilic chromatin. The liquefied nuclear material will be Feulgen-positive as long as it stains a dark violet by panoptic methods.

Disintegrating forms still containing basophilic chromatin are called necrobiotic. If basophilic chromatin is no longer present, they are called necrotic.[174] An excellent set of color plates depicting necrobiosis of blood cells may be found in the *Sandoz Atlas of Hematology*, 2nd ed., Color Plates 409–416.[174]

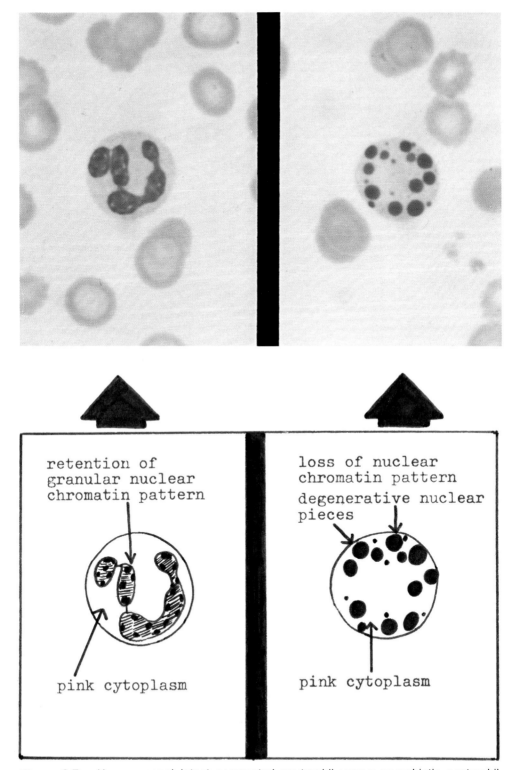

Figure 6.7. *Upper,* normal intact segmented neutrophil *versus* necrobiotic neutrophil. *Lower,* schematic diagram.

The Basophilic Series

Table 6.7
Morphologic Criteria for Basophilic Series
Key Differentiating Feature:
Presence on absence of granules in cell with 3:1 or 4:1 N:C ratio and basophilic cytoplasm.

	Myeloblast	Promyelocyte
Cell size	10–20 μm in diameter	10–20 μm in diameter
Nuclear: cytoplasmic ratio (N:C)	*4:1*	*3:1*
Nuclear shape	Round or oval, slight indentation more commonly seen in leukemic states	Round or oval
Nuclear position	Eccentric or central	Eccentric or central
Nuclear color and chromatin	Light red-purple, fine meshwork with no aggregation of material	Light red-purple, fine meshwork, slight aggregation seen at nuclear rim
Nucleoli	1–5	1–5
Color and amount of cytoplasm	*Basophilic* and scanty	*Basophilic* and slightly increased over myeloblast
Cytoplasmic granules	*Absent*	*Present*, fine azurophilic, nonspecific granules

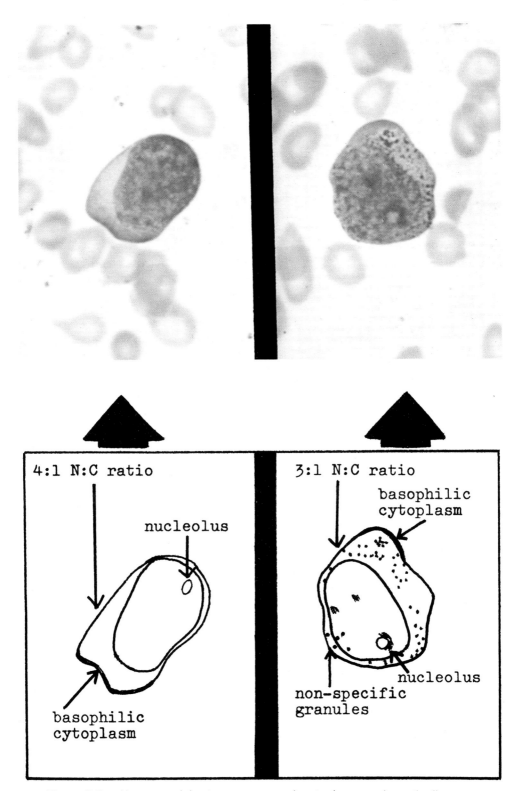

Figure 6.8.   *Upper,* myelobast *versus* promyelocyte. *Lower,* schematic diagram.

Table 6.8
Morphologic Criteria for Basophilic Series
Key Differentiating Feature:
The decrease in the nuclear area coupled to a decrease in basophilia of the cytoplasm and the appearance of large, coarse nonuniform, water-soluble, purple-black granules.

	Promyelocyte	Basophilic Myelocyte
Cell size	10–20 μm in diameter	10–20 μm in diameter
Nuclear: cytoplasmic ratio (N:C)	*3:1*	*2:1 or 1:1*
Nuclear shape	Round or oval	Oval or slightly indented, occasionally round
Nuclear position	Eccentric or central	Commonly eccentric, may be central
Nuclear color and chromatin	Light red-purple fine meshwork, slight aggregation may be seen at nuclear membrane in late stages	Red-purple fine chromatin with slightly aggregated or granular pattern
Nucleoli	1–5	May or may not have nucleolus
Color and amount of cytoplasm	*Basophilic*, slightly increased amount over myeloblast	*Bluish-pale*, moderate
Cytoplasmic granules	Present, *fine azurophilic, nonspecific granules*	Present, *coarse purple-black non-uniform granules* (*water-soluble, may dissolve in staining*)

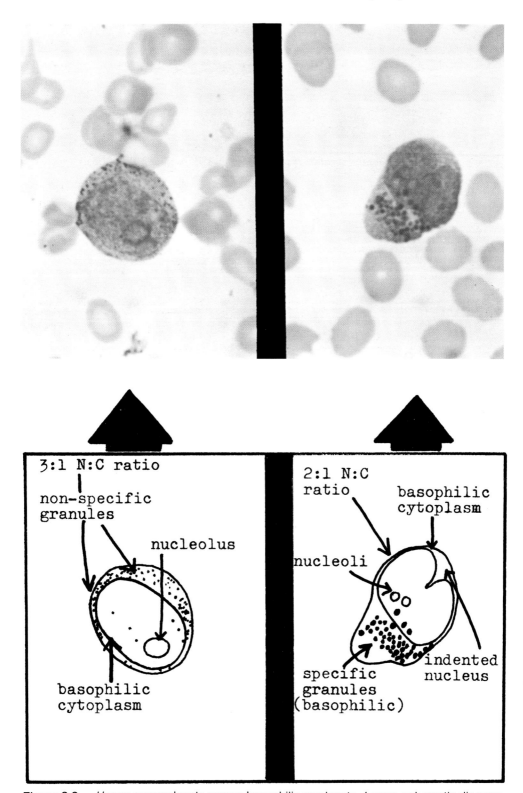

Figure 6.9. *Upper*, promyelocyte *versus* basophilic myelocyte. *Lower*, schematic diagram.

Table 6.9
Morphologic Criteria for Basophilic Series
Key Differentiating Feature:
Change from fine red-purple chromatin to light blue-purple distinct basi- and oxyphilic-chromatin and increased nuclear indentation with coarse purple-black granules.

	Basophilic Myelocyte	Basophilic Metamyelocyte
Cell size	10–18 μm in diameter	10–18 μm in diameter
Nuclear cytoplasmic ratio (N:C)	2:1 or 1:1	1:1
Nuclear shape	*Oval* or slightly indented, occasionally round	*Usually indented, (kidney-shaped)*, oval, and rarely round
Nuclear position	Commonly eccentric, may be central	Central or eccentric
Nuclear color and chromatin	*Red-purple fine chromatin* with slightly aggregated or granular pattern	*Light blue-purple with basi- and oxyphilic chromatin easily distinguishable*
Nucleoli	May or may not have nucleolus	None
Color and amount of cytoplasm	*Bluish-pale*, moderate	*Pale* blue, moderate
Cytoplasmic granules	Present, coarse purple-black nonuniform granules (*water-soluble, may dissolve in staining*)	Present, coarse purple-black nonuniform granules (*water-soluble, may dissolve in staining*)

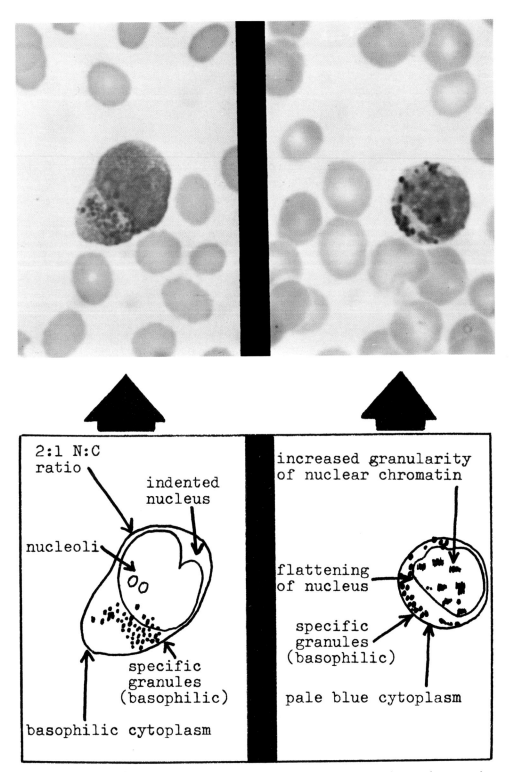

Figure 6.10. *Upper,* basophilic myelocyte *versus* basophilic metamyelocyte. *Lower,* schematic diagram.

Table 6.10
Morphologic Criteria for Basophilic Series
Key Differentiating Feature:
Change from kidney-shaped or wide oval nucleus to narrow elongated band nuclear shape and increased granularity of nucleus with coarse purple-black nonuniform granules.

	Basophilic Metamyelocyte	Basophilic Band
Cell size	10–18 μm in diameter	10–16 μm in diameter
Nuclear: cytoplasmic ratio (N:C)	1:1	1:1
Nuclear shape	*Usually indented, (kidney-shaped), oval, and rarely round*	*Elongated, narrow band shape of uniform thickness singular nuclear lobe*
Nuclear position	Central or eccentric	Central or eccentric
Nuclear color and chromatin	*Light blue-purple with basi- and oxyphilic chromatin easily distinguishable*	*Deep blue-purple coarsely granular chromatin*
Nucleoli	None	None
Color and amount of cytoplasm	Pale blue, moderate	Pale blue, moderate
Cytoplasmic granules	Present, *coarse purple-black nonuniform granules* (water-soluble, may dissolve in staining)	Present *coarse purple-black nonuniform granules* (water-soluble, may dissolve in staining)

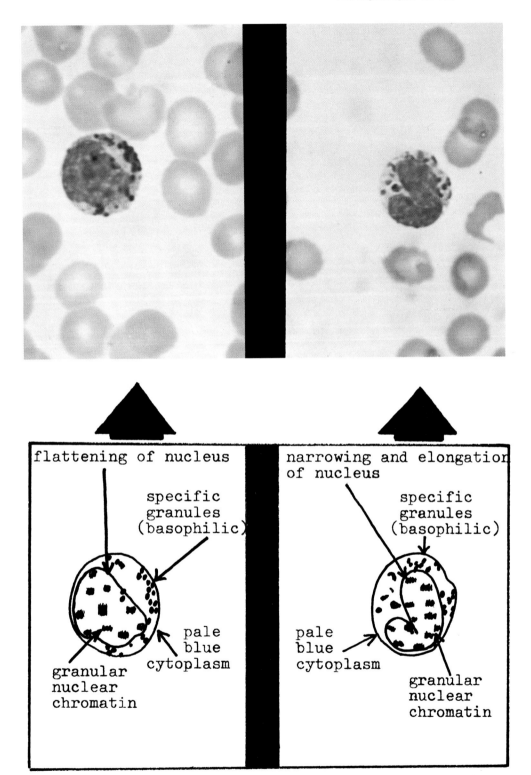

Figure 6.11. *Upper*, basophilic metamyelocyte *versus* basophilic band neutrophil. *Lower*, schematic diagram.

Table 6.11
Morphologic Criteria for Basophilic Series
Key Differentiating Feature:
Change from elongated, narrow singular nuclear lobe to a multilobed (0–4) with coarse purple-black nonuniform granules.

	Basophilic Band	Basophilic Segmented Neutrophil
Cell size	10–16 μm in diameter	10–16 μm in diameter
Nuclear: cytoplasmic ratio (N:C)	1:1	1:1
Nuclear shape	Elongated, narrow band shape of uniform thickness, singular nuclear lobe	0–2 distinct nuclear lobes, rarely 3 or 4 lobes seen (0.5 μm filament connecting lobes)
Nuclear position	Central or eccentric	Central or eccentric
Nuclear color and chromatin	Deep blue-purple coarsely granular chromatin	Deep blue-purple coarsely granular chromatin
Nucleoli	None	None
Color and amount of cytoplasm	Pale blue abundant	Pale blue, abundant
Cytoplasmic granules	Present, coarse purple-black nonuniform granules (water-soluble, may dissolve in staining)	Present coarse purple-black nonuniform granules (water-soluble, may dissolve in staining)

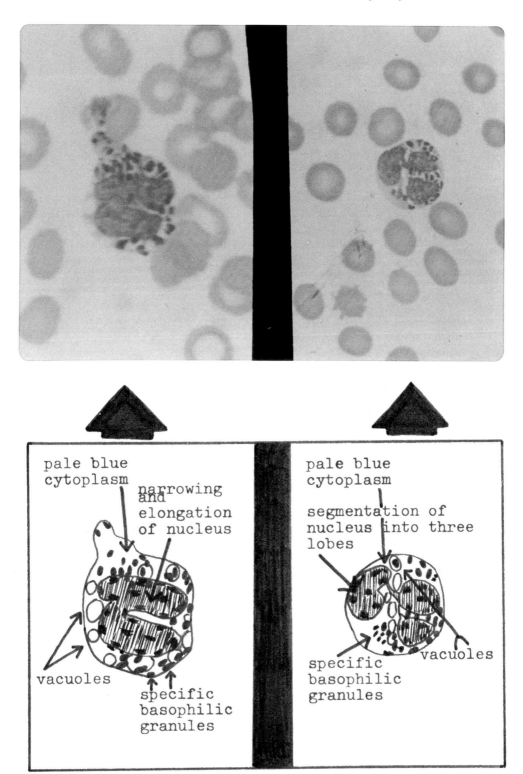

Figure 6.12.   *Upper,* basophilic band neutrophil *versus* basophilic segmented neutrophil. *Lower,* schematic diagram.

The Eosinophilic Series

Table 6.12
Morphologic Criteria for Eosinophilic Series
Key Differentiating Feature:
Presence or absence of granules in cell with 3:1 or 4:1 N:C ratio and basophilic cytoplasm.

	Myeloblast	Promyelocyte
Cell size	10–20 μm in diameter	10–20 μm in diameter
Nuclear: cytoplasmic ratio (N:C)	*4:1*	*3:1*
Nuclear shape	Round or oval, slight indentation more commonly seen in leukemic states	Round or oval
Nuclear position	Eccentric or central	Eccentric or central
Nuclear color and chromatin	Light red-purple, fine meshwork with no aggregation of material	Light red-purple, fine meshwork, slight aggregation may be seen at nuclear membrane
Nucleoli	1–5	1–5
Color and amount of cytoplasm	*Basophilic* and scanty	*Basophilic* and slightly increased over myeloblast
Cytoplasmic granules	*Absent*	*Present, fine azurophilic, nonspecific granules*

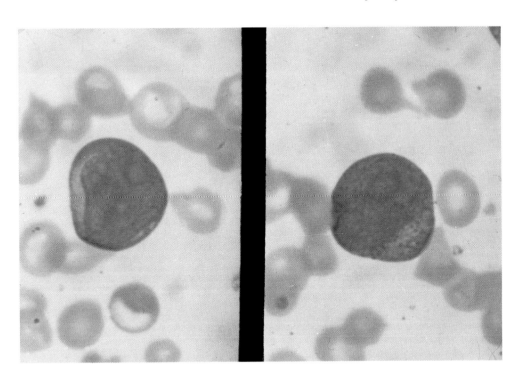

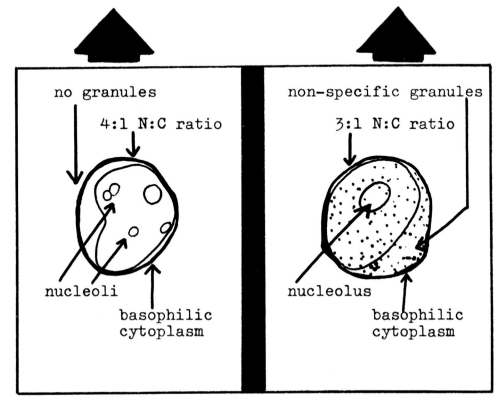

Figure 6.13. *Upper*, myeloblast *versus* promyelocyte. *Lower*, schematic diagram.

Table 6.13
Morphologic Criteria for Eosinophilic Series
Key Differentiating Feature:
The decrease in the nuclear area coupled to a decrease in basophilia of the cytoplasm and the appearance of large, red specific eosinophilic granules.

	Promyelocyte	Eosinophilic Myelocyte
Cell size	10–20 μm in diameter	10–18 μm in diameter
Nuclear: cytoplasmic ratio (N:C)	*3:1*	*2:1 or 1:1*
Nuclear shape	Round or oval	Oval or slightly indented, occasionally round
Nuclear position	Eccentric or central	Commonly eccentric may be central
Nuclear color and chromatin	Light red-purple, fine meshwork, slight aggregation may be seen at nuclear membrane in late stages	Red-purple fine chromatin with slightly aggregated or granular pattern
Nucleoli	1–5	May or may not have nucleolus
Color and amount of cytoplasm	*Basophilic*, slightly increased amount over myeloblast	*Bluish-pink*, moderate
Cytoplasmic granules	Present, fine azurophilic, *nonspecific granules*	Present, *red, uniform specific granules* (*eosinophilic*)

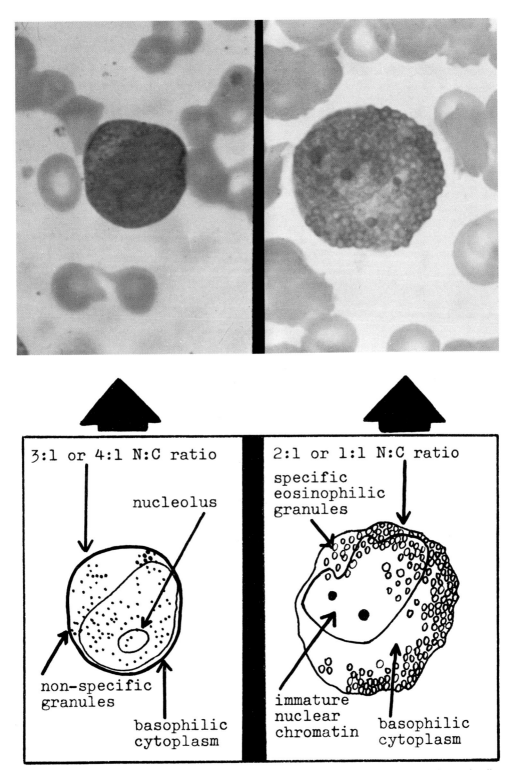

Figure 6.14. *Upper,* promyelocyte *versus* eosinophilic myelocyte. *Lower,* schematic diagram.

Table 6.14
Morphologic Criteria for Eosinophilic Series
Key Differentiating Feature:
Changes from fine red-purple chromatin to light blue-purple distinct basi-
and oxyphilic chromatin and increased nuclear indentation with red
granules.

	Eosinophilic Myelocyte	Eosinophilic Metamyelo-cyte
Cell size	10–18 μm in diameter	10–18 μm in diameter
Nuclear: cytoplasmic ratio (N:C)	2:1 or 1:1	1:1
Nuclear shape	*Oval* or slightly indented, occasionally round	*Usually indented* (*kidney-shaped*), oval, and rarely round
Nuclear position	Commonly eccentric may be central	Central or eccentric
Nuclear color and chromatin	*Red-purple fine chromatin with* slightly aggregated or granular pattern	*Light blue-purple with basi- and oxyphilic chromatin easily distinguishable*
Nucleoli	May or may not have nucleolus	None
Color and amount of cytoplasm	*Bluish-pink*, moderate	*Pink*, moderate
Cytoplasmic granules	Present, red, uniform specific granules (eosinophilic)	Present, red, uniform specific granules (eosinophilic)

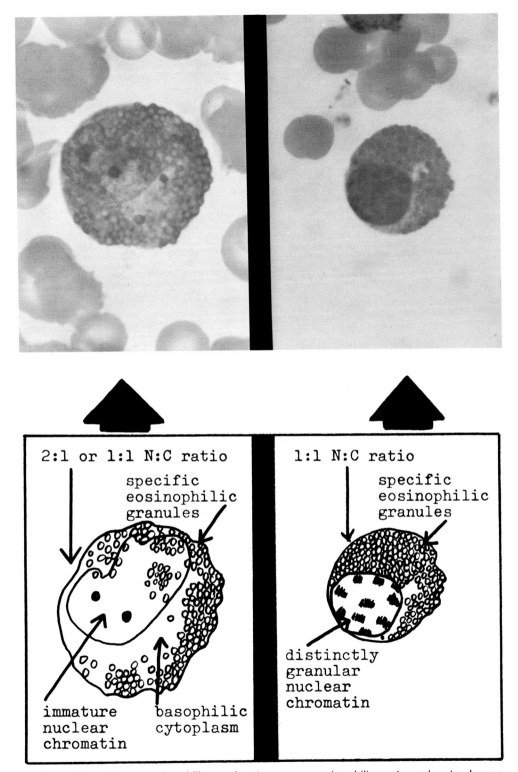

Figure 6.15. *Upper,* eosinophilic myelocyte *versus* eosinophilic metamyelocyte. *Lower,* schematic diagram.

Table 6.15
Morphologic Criteria for Eosinophilic Series
Key Differentiating Feature:
Change from kidney-shaped or wide oval nucleus to narrow elongated band nuclear shape and increased nuclear granularity with red uniform granules.

	Eosinophilic Metamyelocyte	Eosinophilic Band Neutrophil
Cell size	10–18 μm in diameter	10–16 μm in diameter
Nuclear: cytoplasmic ratio (N:C)	1:1	1:1
Nuclear shape	*Usually indented, (kidney-shaped), oval, and rarely round*	*Elongated, narrow band shape of uniform thickness singular nuclear lobe*
Nuclear position	Central or eccentric	Central or eccentric
Nuclear color and chromatin	*Light blue-purple with basi- and oxyphilic chromatin easily distinguishable*	*deep blue-purple coarsely granular chromatin*
Nucleoli	None	None
Color and amount of cytoplasm	Pink, moderate	Pink, abundant
Cytoplasmic granules	Present, red, uniform specific granules (eosinophilic)	Present, red, uniform specific granules (eosinophilic)

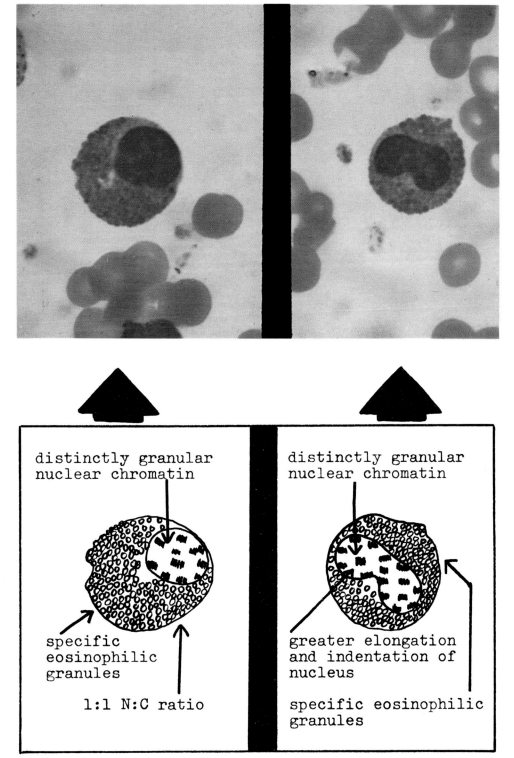

Figure 6.16. *Upper,* eosinophilic metamyelocyte *versus* eosinophilic band neutrophil. *Lower,* schematic diagram.

Table 6.16
Morphologic Criteria for Eosinophilic Series
Key Differentiating Feature:
Change from elongated narrow singular nuclear lobe to a multilobed (0–2) (rarely 3–4 lobes) with red, uniform granules.

	Eosinophilic Band Neutrophil	Eosinophilic Segmented Neutrophil
Cell size	10–16 μm in diameter	10–16 μm in diameter
Nuclear: cytoplasmic ratio (N:C)	1:1	1:1
Nuclear shape	*Elongated, narrow band shape of uniform thickness, singular nuclear lobe*	*0–2 distinct nuclear lobes, rarely 3 or 4 lobes seen (0.5 μm filament connecting lobes)*
Nuclear position	Central or eccentric	Central or eccentric
Nuclear color and chromatin	Deep blue-purple coarsely granular chromatin	Deep blue-purple coarsely granular chromatin
Nucleoli	None	None
Color and amount of cytoplasm	Pink, abundant	Pink, abundant
Cytoplasmic granules	Present, red, uniform specific granules (eosinophilic)	Present, red, uniform specific granules (eosinophilic)

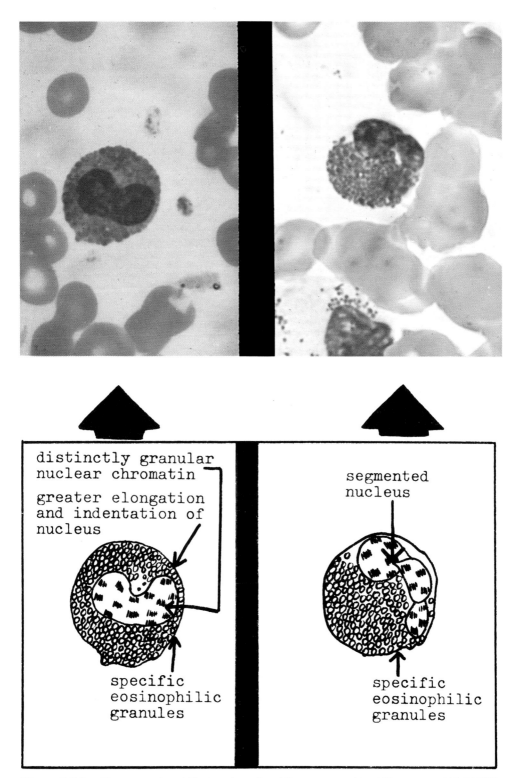

Figure 6.17. *Upper*, eosinophilic band neutrophil *versus* eosinophilic segmented neutrophil. *Lower*, schematic diagram.

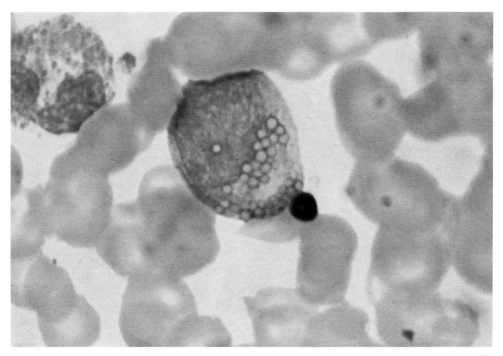

Figure 6.18.   Abnormal immature eosinophilic myelocyte (original magnification ×1500).

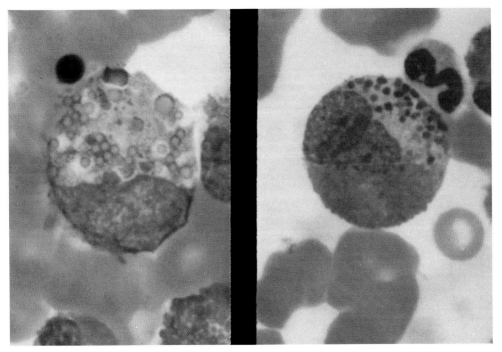

Figure 6.19.   See legend, Figure 6.18.

Chapter 7

The Plasmacytic Series

Table 7.1
Morphologic Criteria for Plasmacytic Series
Key Differentiating Feature:
Change from fine, stippled nuclear chromatin to increased granularity of
pattern and increase in basophilia of cytoplasm.

	Plasmablast	Proplasmacyte
Cell size	16–18 μm in diameter	15–25 μm in diameter
Nuclear:cytoplasmic ratio (N:C)	4:1	3:1
Nuclear shape	Round	Round or oval
Nuclear position	Central or eccentric	Central or eccentric
Nuclear color and chromatin	Pale red-purple, *fine stippled chromatin*	Red-purple, *increased granularity of chromatin*
Nucleoli	Usually 1–3	Usually 1–3
Color and amount of cytoplasm	Scanty to moderate, *paler blue* than more mature forms occasionally perinuclear clear zone	Moderate, *basophilic*, may or may not have perinuclear clear zone adjacent to the nucleus
Cytoplasmic granules	None	None

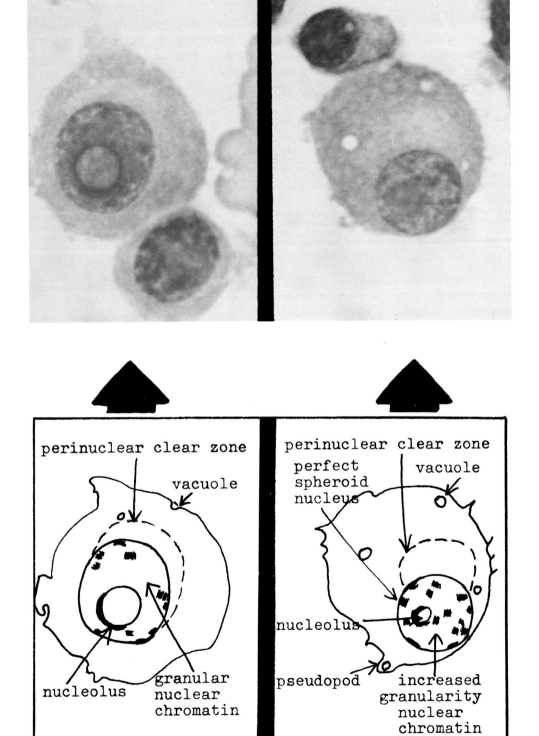

Figure 7.1 *Upper*, Plasmablast *versus* proplasmacyte. *Lower*, schematic diagram.

Table 7.2
Morphologic Criteria for Plasmacytic Series
Key Differentiating Feature:
Change from red-purple to blue-purple denser, more granular nuclear chromatin in slightly smaller cell.

	Proplasmacyte	Mature Plasma Cell
Cell size	*15–25 μm* in diameter	*8–20 μm* in diameter
Nuclear:cytoplasmic ratio (N:C)	3:1	2:1 or 1:1
Nuclear shape	Round or oval	Round or oval
Nuclear position	Central or eccentric	Frequently eccentric, occasionally may be central
Nuclear color and chromatin	*Red-purple, increased granularity of chromatin*	*Blue-purple, dense chromatin with large clumps near nuclear margin*
Nucleoli	Usually 1–3	None
Color and amount of cytoplasm	Moderate basophilic, may or may not have perinuclear clear zone adjacent to the nucleus	Moderate, basophilic, with perinuclear clear zone adjacent to nucleus, may contain one or more vacuoles
Cytoplasmic granules	None	None

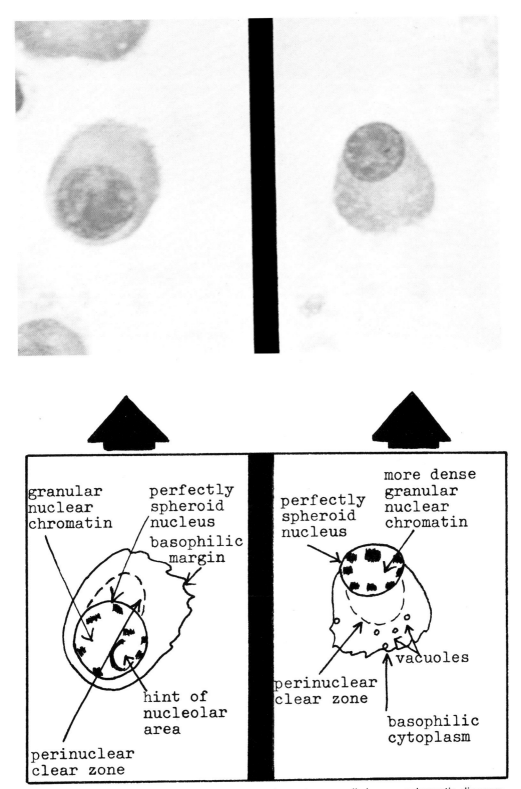

Figure 7.2. *Upper,* proplasmacyte *versus* mature plasma cell. *Lower,* schematic diagram.

Chapter 8

The Lymphocytic Series

Table 8.1
Morphologic Criteria for Lymphocytic Series
Key Differentiating Feature:
Change from undifferentiated nuclear chromatin to the combined blue-purple, red-purple chromatin-parachromatin giving light-dark effect to nucleus.

	Lymphoblast	Immature Lymphocyte
Cell size	10–20 μm in diameter	9–18 μm in diameter
Nuclear: cytoplasmic ratio (N:C)	4:1	4:1 (occasionally 3:1
Nuclear shape	Round or oval	Round or indented
Nuclear position	Eccentric or central	Eccentric with scanty cytoplasm to one side or round
Nuclear color and chromatin	*Undifferentiated, sparse red-purple chromatin*	*Combination of condensed clumped blue-purple chromatin with red-purple parachromatin (light and dark)*
Nucleoli	1–2	0–1, less distinct
Color and amount of cytoplasm	Scanty, clear basophilic	Scanty, clear basophilic
Cytoplasmic granules	Absent	Absent

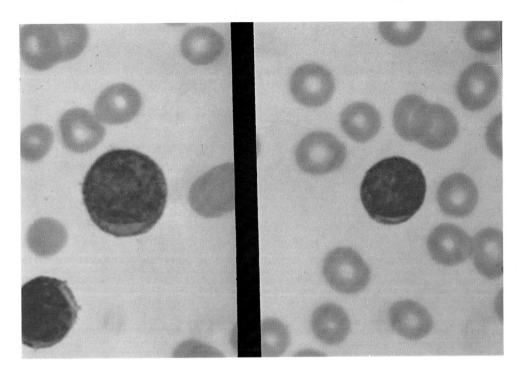

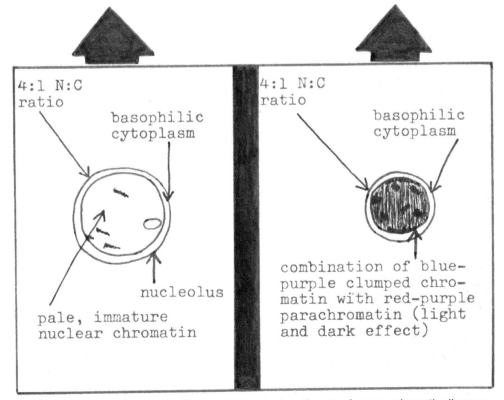

Figure 8.1   *Upper*, lymphoblast *versus* immature lymphocyte. *Lower*, schematic diagram.

Table 8.2
Morphologic Criteria for Lymphocytic Series
Key Differentiating Feature:
Loss of visible red-purple parachromatin from nucleus and change in cytoplasmic color from basophilic to skyblue.

	Immature lymphocyte	Mature Lymphocyte
Cell size	9–18 μm in diameter	7–18 μm in diameter (most forms 9–12 μm in diameter)
Nuclear: cytoplasmic ratio (:C)	4:1 (occasionally 3:1	4:1 (occasionally 3:1)
Nuclear shape	Round or indented	Round or indented
Nuclear position	Eccentric with scanty cytoplasm to one side or round	Eccentric with scanty cytoplasm to one side or round
Nuclear color and chromatin	*Combination of condensed clumped blue-purple chromatin with red-purple parachromatin (light and dark)*	*Homogenous, coarse blue-purple nuclear chromatin*
Nucleoli	0–1, less distinct	Usually absent, rarely one seen in mature form
Color and amount of cytoplasm	Scanty, clear *basophilic*	*Light clear sky blue*, scanty to moderate
Cytoplasmic granules	Absent	Usually absent, occasionally few azurophilic granules seen

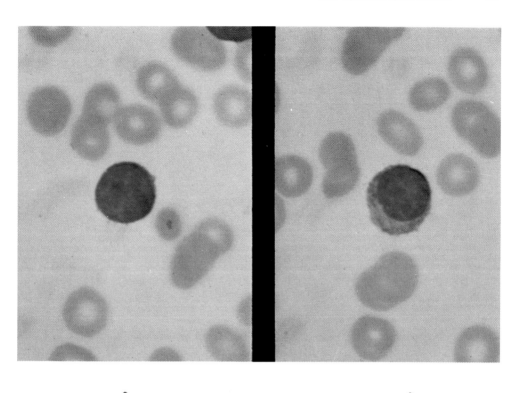

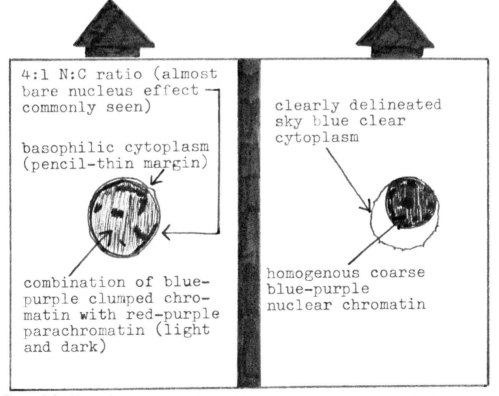

4:1 N:C ratio (almost
bare nucleus effect
commonly seen)

basophilic cytoplasm
(pencil-thin margin)

combination of blue-
purple clumped chro-
matin with red-purple
parachromatin (light
and dark)

clearly delineated
sky blue clear
cytoplasm

homogenous coarse
blue-purple
nuclear chromatin

Figure 8.2 *Upper*, immature lymphocyte *versus* lymphocyte. *Lower*, schematic diagram.

Atypical Lymphocytes

Atypical lymphocytes have been most closely associated with infectious mononucleosis since Downey's classic division of these cells into three types in 1923.[55] The atypical lymphocytes seen in infectious mononucleosis, however, cannot be distinguished from those seen in a variety of viral diseases, for example, infectious hepatitis, chickenpox, cytomegalovirus, etc. Their association with viral disease inspired Litwins and Leibowitz in 1951 to call them "virocytes."[59] This term is not all inclusive though, since they may also be seen in normal persons and in patients with a drug hypersensitivity. Downey's three categories are considered by some investigators to be obsolete and of little practical importance. These cells are the core of much controversy among hematologists.

However, from a teaching viewpoint, Downey's descriptions have been most helpful in delineating the morphological differences in these cells for students and I feel that the vast majority of these atypical lymphocytes do fit into one of his original categories.

The student should keep in mind that these are highly differentiated mature reactive lymphocytes and they differ from their immature counterparts (lymphoblasts and young lymphocytes) in two ways: 1) atypical lymphocytes contain mature coarse red-purple nuclear chromatin in contrast to immature forms which contain pale-staining immature nuclear chromatin with large amounts of parachromatin; and 2) atypical lymphocytes possess abundant cytoplasm, not scanty as in immature forms.

ATYPICAL LYMPHOCYTES SEEN IN INFECTIOUS MONONUCLEOSIS

All of the color plates of Downey-type atypical lymphocytes on page 91 were taken from the same peripheral blood smear of a 24-year-old patient with infectious mononucleosis.

Figure 8.3. Normal lymphocyte.
Figure 8.4. *A, B,* and *C,* Downey type I atypical lymphocyte. Slightly indented nucleus with increased granularity of chromatin reminiscent of a plasma cell; however, most chromatin retains the dense, homogenous pattern of the mature lymphocyte. Cytoplasm is vacuolated and foamy, may be one-sided, and is usually basophilic in color.
Figure 8.5. *A, B,* and *C,* Downey type II atypical lymphocyte. Coarse dense nuclear chromatin but not as condensed as Downey Type I with one or more nucleoli. Cytoplasm is not as foamy as Type I. It has a frequently irregular border (scalloped effect) which may flow around adjacent rbcs. Cytoplasm is usually pale blue with a deeper blue at the extreme border. Azurophilic granules are occasionally seen.
Figure 8.6. *A, B,* and *C,* Downey Type III atypical lymphocyte. Coarse clumped red-purple nuclear chromatin with one to four nucleoli. Nucleus commonly appears to be stretched the length of the cell. Abundant, deeply basophilic cytoplasm with an irregular border frequently and the tendency to flow around adjacent rbcs.

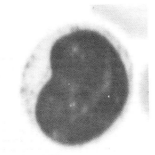

Figure 8.3

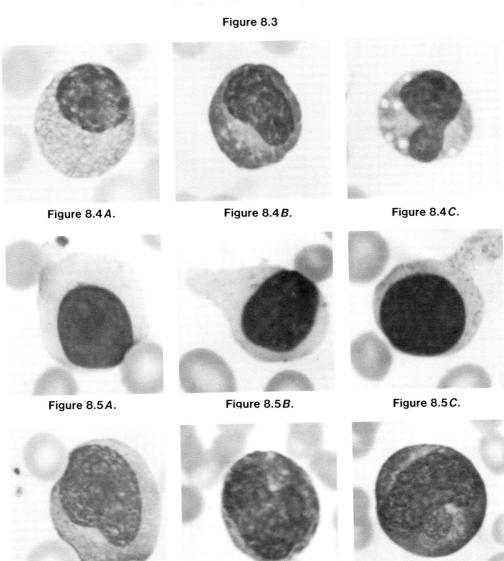

Figure 8.4 A.

Figure 8.4 B.

Figure 8.4 C.

Figure 8.5 A.

Figure 8.5 B.

Figure 8.5 C.

Figure 8.6 A.

Figure 8.6 B.

Figure 8.6 C.

Chapter 9

The Monocytic Series

Table 9.1
Morphologic Criteria for Monocytic Series
Key Differentiating Feature:
Change from homogenous unidentified nuclear chromatin to reticular pattern with creases or folds and change from darker basophilic cytoplasm to pale grey blue with irregular borders.

	Monoblast	Immature Monocytes
Cell size	12–20 μm in diameter	12–20 μm in diameter
Nuclear: cytoplasmic ratio (N:C)	4:1	3:1 or 2:1
Nuclear shape	Round, oval, or *slightly folded*	Round with *chromatin creases* or *cerebriform folding, more distinct*
Nuclear position	Central	Central
Nuclear color and chromatin	Pale red-purple, *minimal, fine, thready chromatin*	Pale red-purple, *reticular pattern (aerated network of threads) very fine*
Nucleoli	Usually 1–2, occasionally 3 or 4	0–2
Color and amount of cytoplasm	*Basophilic*, moderate, regular border	*Paler gray-basophilia, more abundant, equally proportioned around nucleus with "bleblike" pseudopodia at border*
Cytoplasmic granules	*None*	*May or may not contain fine red dust-like particles*

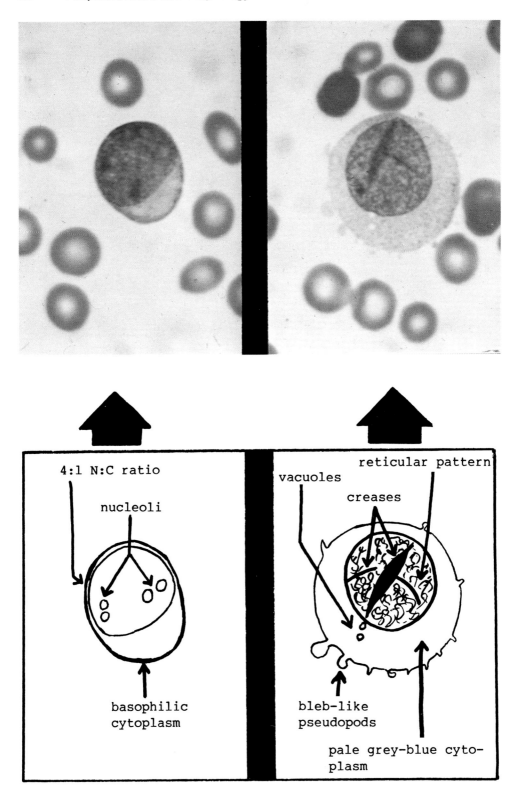

Figure 9.1.1. *Upper*, Monoblast *versus* immature monocyte. *Lower*, schematic diagram.

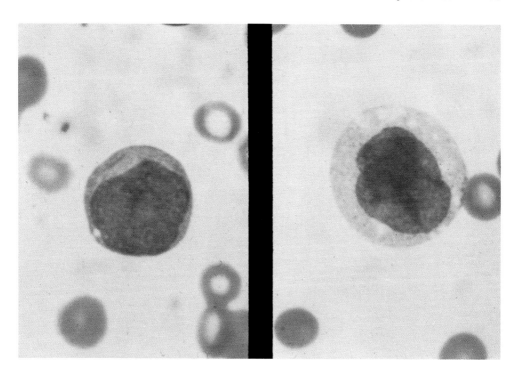

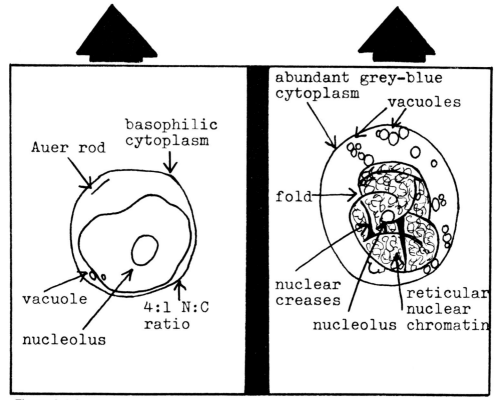

Figure 9.1.2. *Upper*, monoblast *versus* immature monocyte. *Lower*, schematic diagram.

Table 9.2
Morphologic Criteria for Monocytic Series
Key Differentiating Feature:
The increased folding and finer blue-purple reticular pattern of the nucleus coupled to the paler gray-blue of the cytoplasm. Loss of nucleoli in some forms.

	Immature Monocytes	Mature Monocytes
Cell size	12–20 μm in diameter	12–20 μm in diameter
Nuclear: cytoplasmic ratio (N:C)	3:1 or 2:1	2:1 or 1:1
Nuclear shape	*Round with chromatin creases or cerebriform, folding,* more distinct than monoblast	*Increased folding (cerebriform) or narrow, elongated (horseshoe shape)*
Nuclear position	Central	Central
Nuclear color and chromatin	Pale *red-purple reticular pattern (aerated network of threads) very fine*	*Blue-purple, finer reticular pattern than immature forms*
Nucleoli	*0–2*	*None*
Color and amount of cytoplasm	Paler *gray, basophilia* more abundant, equally proportioned round nucleus with "bleb-like" pseudopodia at border	Abundant *pale gray-blue, lighter than immature forms,* equally proportioned round the nucleus ("bleb-like" pseudopodia)
Cytoplasmic granules	May or may not contain fine red dust-like particles	*More numerous fine pale red dust-like particles evenly dispersed*

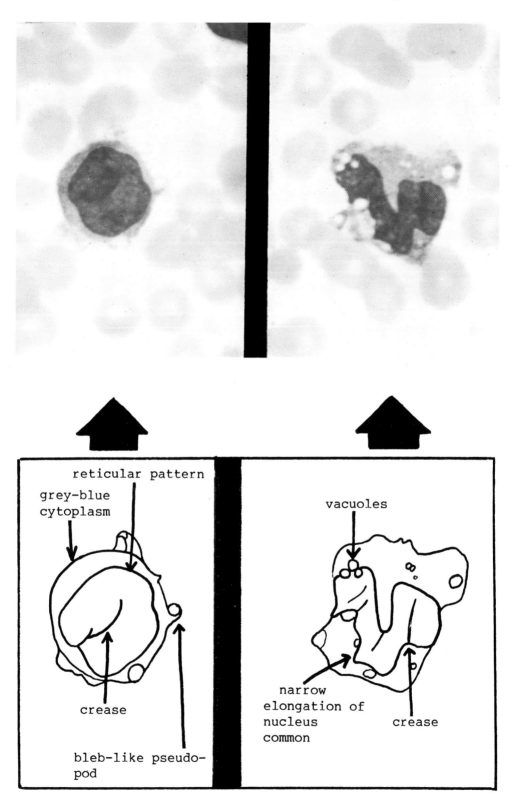

Figure 9.2. *Upper*, immature monocyte *versus* mature monocyte. *Lower*, schematic diagram.

Chapter 10

The Megakaryocytic Series

Table 10.1
Morphologic Criteria for Megakaryocytic Series
Key Differentiating Feature:
Increased granularity of nuclear chromatin coupled to appearance of azurophilic granules in cytoplasm. Increment of granules and cytoplasm as cell matures.

	Megakaryoblast	Promegakaryocyte
Cell size	15–50 μm in diameter	20–80 μm in diameter
Nuclear: cytoplasmic ratio (N:C)	*4:1*	*4:1–1:1*
Nuclear shape	Usually single round, oval, indented or kidney-shaped (multinucleated forms rarely seen)	Usually single round, oval, indented or kidney-shaped (rarely multinucleated forms)
Nuclear position	Central or eccentric	Central or eccentric
Nuclear color and chromatin	*Red-purple fine chromatin with distinct "smudged" chromatin clumps*	*Red-purple, increased granularity of nuclear chromatin*
Nucleoli	1–5	Usually less numerous than megakaryoblast but may be as numerous (1–5)
Color and amount of cytoplasm	Varying shades of blue, usually basophilic, amount varies from narrow rim to abundant with pseudopodia frequently	Usually abundant with pseudopodia frequently, usually basophilic, but paler as maturity approaches
Cytoplasmic granules	*Usually absent rarely few granules (azurophilic) may be seen*	*Fine azurophilic granules most abundant adjacent to the nucleus*

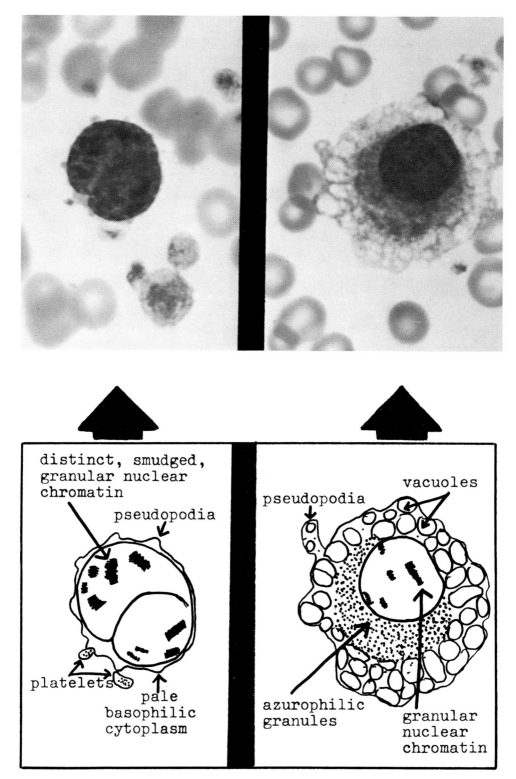

Figure 10.1. *Upper,* megakaryoblast *versus* promegakaryocyte. *Lower,* schematic diagram.

Table 10.2
Morphologic Criteria for Megakaryocytic Series
Key Differentiating Feature:
Appearance of lobulated nuclear shape and markedly increased complement of cytoplasm.

	Promegakaryocyte	Megakaryocyte
Cell size	20–80 μm in diameter	35–160 μm in diameter
Nuclear: cytoplasmic ratio (N:C)	4:1–1:1	1:1–1:12
Nuclear shape	*Usually single, round, oval, indented or kidney-shaped (rarely multinucleated forms)*	*Lobulated (2 or more lobes)*
Nuclear position	Central or eccentric	Central
Nuclear color and chromatin	*Red-purple* increased granularity of nuclear chromatin	*Blue-purple*, granular
Nucleoli	Usually less numerous than megakaryoblast but may be as numerous (1–5)	None
Color and amount of cytoplasm	Usually abundant with pseudopodia frequently— *usually basophilic* but paler as maturity approaches	*Abundant pale blue* (with pink cast) may exhibit pseudopodia
Cytoplasmic granules	Fine azurophilic granules, most abundant adjacent to the nucleus	*Numerous* fine azurophilic granules evenly distributed

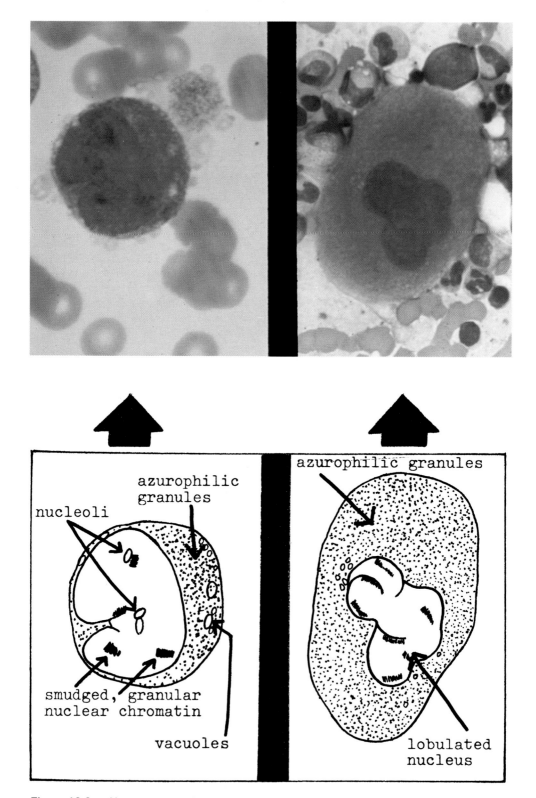

Figure 10.2.   *Upper*, promegakaryocyte *versus* megakaryocyte. *Lower*, schematic diagram.

Table 10.3
Morphologic Criteria for Megakaryocytic Series
Key Differentiating Feature:
Loss of nucleus and reduction of cytoplasmic area to small fragment.

	Megakaryocyte	Thrombocyte (Platelet)
Cell size	35–160 μm in diameter	2–4 μm in diameter
Nuclear: cytoplasmic ratio (N:C)	1:1–1:2	—
Nuclear shape	*Lobulated* (2 or more lobes)	—
Nuclear position		—
Nuclear color and chromatin	Blue-purple granular	—
Nucleoli	None	—
Color and amount of cytoplasm	Abundant pale blue (with pink cast) may exhibit pseudopodia	Light blue (hyalomere), *fragment of megakaryocyte cytoplasm*
Cytoplasmic granules	Numerous fine azurophilic granules, evenly distributed	Evenly dispersed, fine red-purple granules (chromomere of granulomete)

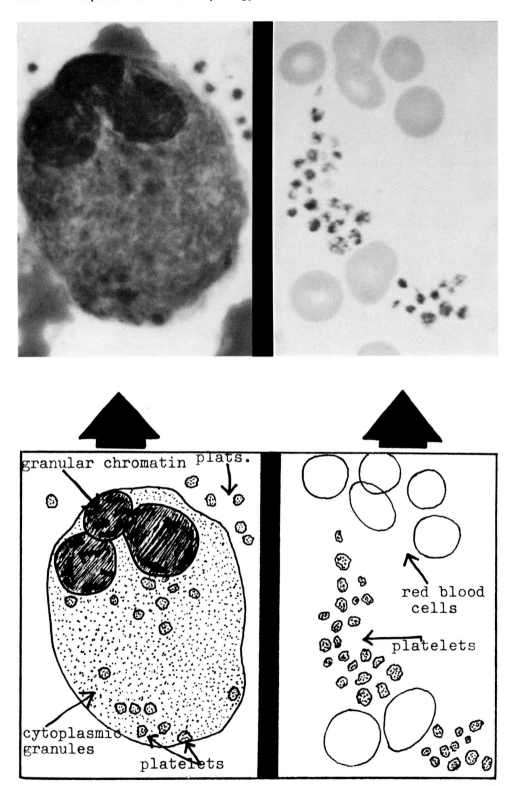

Figure 10.3.   *Upper*, megakaryocyte *versus* thrombocytes (platelets). *Lower*, schematic diagram.

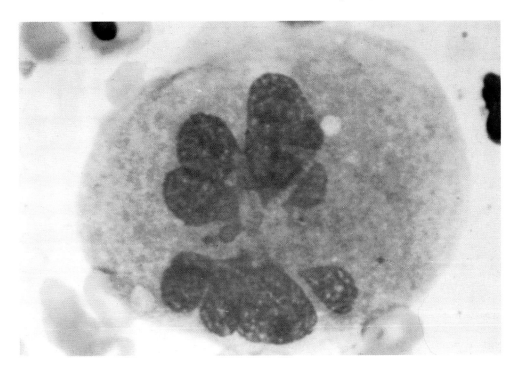

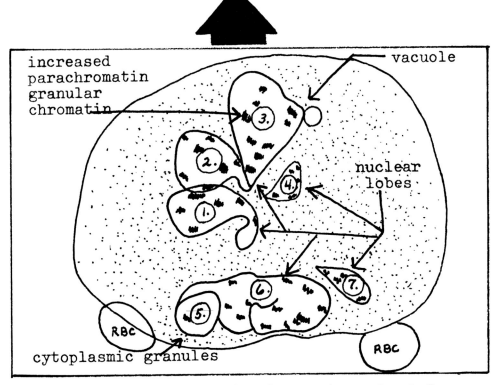

increased
parachromatin
granular
chromatin

vacuole

nuclear
lobes

RBC

cytoplasmic granules

RBC

Figure 10.4. *Upper*, hypersegmented megakaryocyte. *Lower*, schematic diagram.

Table 10.4
Platelets

Criteria	Normal	Abnormal
Size	2–4 μm	5 μm or greater
Cytoplasm	Hyaline, light blue	Increased basophilia or hyaline, light blue
Granules	Evenly dispersed, fine blue-purple type	Tendency to aggregate and/or decreased or absent
Shape	Discoid, oval, or elliptical	May be same as normal but greater tendency to pseudopod formation and bizarre shapes
Vacuoles	None	Not infrequently

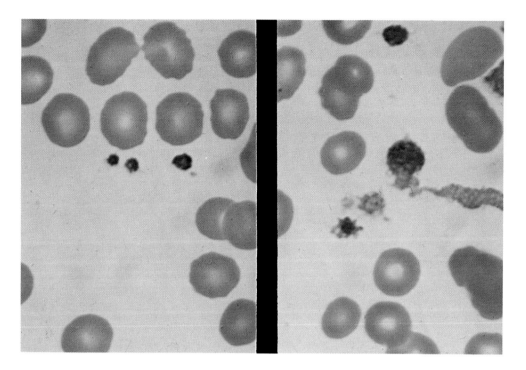

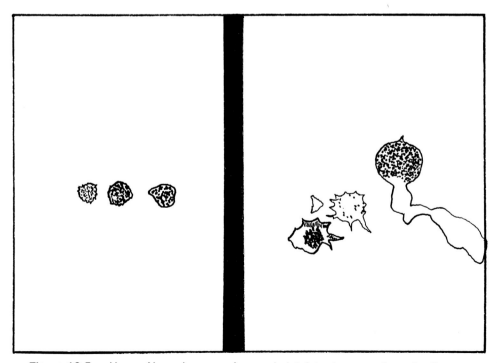

Figure 10.5.   *Upper*, Normal *versus* abnormal platelets. *Lower*, schematic diagram.

Abnormal Morphologic Characteristics of Platelets

1. *Increased size*: 5µ or greater.
2. *Increased basophilia of cytoplasmic membrane.*
3. *Aggregation of granules* (may stimulate pseudo-nucleus).
4. *Absent or decreased granules.*
5. *Pseudopod formation* (bizarre shapes).
6. *Vacuolization of cytoplasmic membrane.*

The presence of any *one* or more of the above named morphologic characteristics in a single platelet constitutes abnormality and should be noted as such.

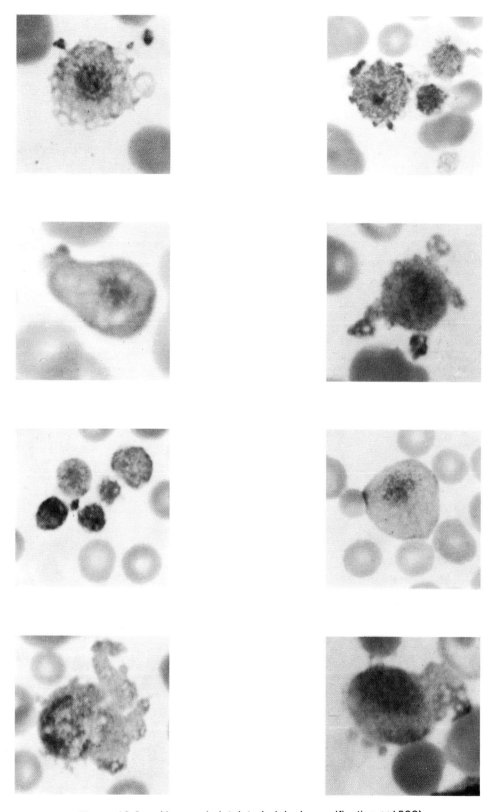

Figure 10.6.   Abnormal platelets (original magnification ×1500).

Platelet Satellitosis

Peripheral blood smears occasionally reveal platelets adhering to neutrophils in a satellite formation as well as actual phagocytosis of these platelets. Rarely, monocytes exhibit platelet phagocytosis as well. McDonald *et al.* illustrate satellitosis in their *Atlas of Hematology*.[121] Ravel and Bassart[143] feel that incubation of blood in EDTA enhances satellitosis, but it is not essential to its occurrence. In one psychology patient at the Farmington Medical Center, platelet satellitosis was abundant on manual "wedge" type slides repeatedly but when the technologist made several smears with the "spread" slide technique that is used in our laboratory at Yale-New Haven Hospital from the blood of this same patient, platelet satellitosis was barely apparent and may explain why in our large volume hematology laboratory we have not observed this phenomenon. Ravel and Bassart[143] investigated the possible etiology of platelet satellitosis in seven patients over a 2-year period. They found the satellitosis in finger-puncture capillary blood smears of two of their patients, which eliminated any possibility of artefact being produced by EDTA. In their 50 control patient smears from EDTA-preserved blood, none exhibited satellitosis or phagocytosis. Silbergeit[163] studied platelet-leukocyte aggregation by incubating blood and EDTA for 45 minutes, then adding a small amount of strontium chloride and incubating for 1 hour. He observed various patterns of platelet-leukocyte aggregation of which satellitosis was one variant. Platelet-leukocyte aggregation by this technique was thought to be frequent in patients with intravascular thrombosis. Ravel and Bassart[143] also felt that a tendency toward thrombus formation might contribute to platelet satellitosis but that more evidence is needed to validate or disprove this possibility.

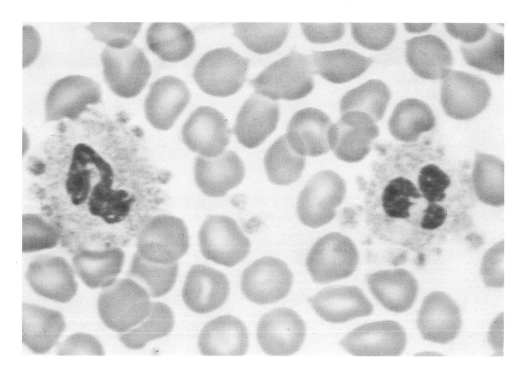

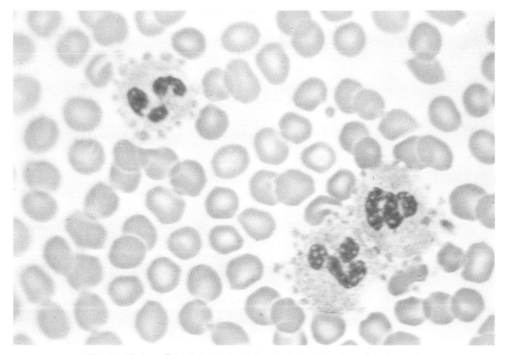

Figure 10.7.   Platelet satellitosis (original magnification ×600).

Chapter 11

The Rubricytic Series

Table 11.1
Morphologic Criteria for Rubricytic Series
Key Differentiating Feature:
The increased granularity of nuclear chromatin and loss of nucleoli in slightly smaller cell.

	Rubriblast	Prorubricyte
Cell size	14–19 μm in diameter	12–17 μm in diameter
Nuclear: cytoplasmic ratio (N:C)	4:1	4:1
Nuclear shape	Round	Round
Nuclear position	Central	Central
Nuclear color and chromatin	Red-purple finely stippled, granular chromatin	*Increased, larger granularity of nuclear chromatin*
Nucleoli	0–2	*Usually none*, occasional cell may show indistinct nucleolus
Color and amount of cytoplasm	Basophilic	Basophilic
Cytoplasmic granules	None	None

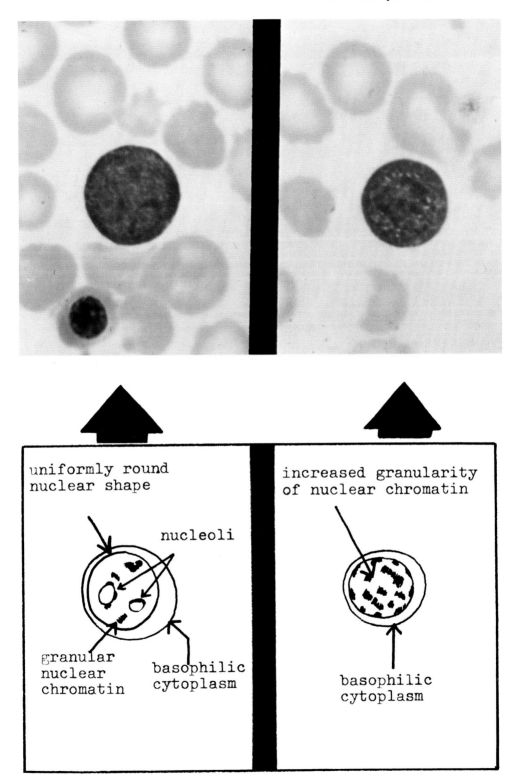

Figure 11.1. *Upper*, rubriblast *versus* prorubricyte. *Lower*, schematic diagram.

Table 11.2
Morphologic Criteria for Rubricytic Series
Key Differentiating Feature:
Increased condensation of nuclear chromatin in smaller nucleus and change in cytoplasmic color to polychromatophilic.

	Prorubricyte	Rubricyte
Cell size	12–17 μm in diameter	12–15 μm in diameter
Nuclear: cytoplasmic ratio (N:C)	4:1	4:1
Nuclear shape	Round	Round
Nuclear position	Central	Central
Nuclear color and chromatin	Increased larger granularity of nuclear chromatin	Red-purple, *smaller nucleus with increased condensation of chromatin*
Nucleoli	Usually none, occasional cell may show indistinct nucleolus	None
Color and amount of cytoplasm	*Basophilic*	Moderate amount, *polychromato-philic*, may contain pink areas of hemoglobin near nucleus
Cytoplasmic granules	None	None

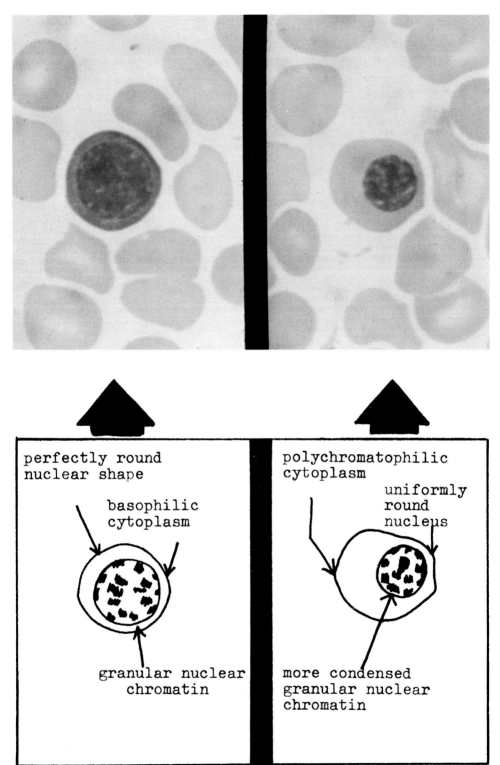

Figure 11.2. *Upper*, prorubricyte *versus* rubricyte. *Lower*, schematic diagram.

Table 11.3
Morphologic Criteria for Rubricytic Series
Key Differentiating Feature:
Red-purple to blue-purple nuclear chromatin in still smaller nucleus and change to pyknotic homogenous pattern plus polychromatophilic cytoplasm changes to acidophilic.

	Rubricyte	Metarubricyte
Cell size	12–15 μm in diameter	8–12 μm in diameter
Nuclear: cytoplasmic ratio (N:C)	1:1	1:1
Nuclear shape	Round	Round
Nuclear position	Central	Central
Nuclear color and chromatin	*Red-purple*, smaller nucleus with increased condensation of chromatin	*Blue-purple, still smaller nucleus with pyknotic degeneration and condensed homogenous chromatin*
Nucleoli	None	None
Color and amount of cytoplasm	Moderate amount, *polychromato-philic*, may contain pink areas of hemoglobin near nucleus	Moderate amount, *acidophilic* (*pink*) due to hemoglobin pigment
Cytoplasmic granules	None	None

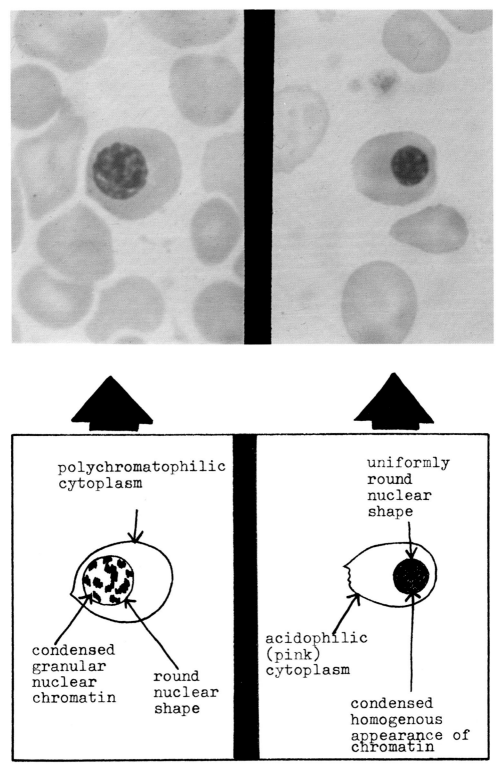

Figure 11.3. *Upper*, rubricyte *versus* metarubricyte. *Lower*, schematic diagram.

Table 11.4
Morphologic Criteria for Rubricytic Series
Key Differentiating Feature:
Loss of nucleus and lessening of cell size and polychromatophilic appearance of cytoplasm in nonnucleated cell.

	Metarubricyte	Polychromatophilic Erythrocyte
Cell size	8–12 μm in diameter	7–10 μm in diameter
Nuclear: cytoplasmic ratio (N:C)	1:1	—
Nuclear shape	Round	—
Nuclear position	Central	—
Nuclear color and chromatin	Blue-purple, still smaller nucleus with pyknotic degeneration and condensed homogenous chromatin	—
Nucleoli	None	—
Color and amount of cytoplasm	Moderate amount, *acidophilic* (pink) due to hemoglobin pigment	Clear gray-blue, *polychromatophilic* to pink
Cytoplasmic granules	None	None

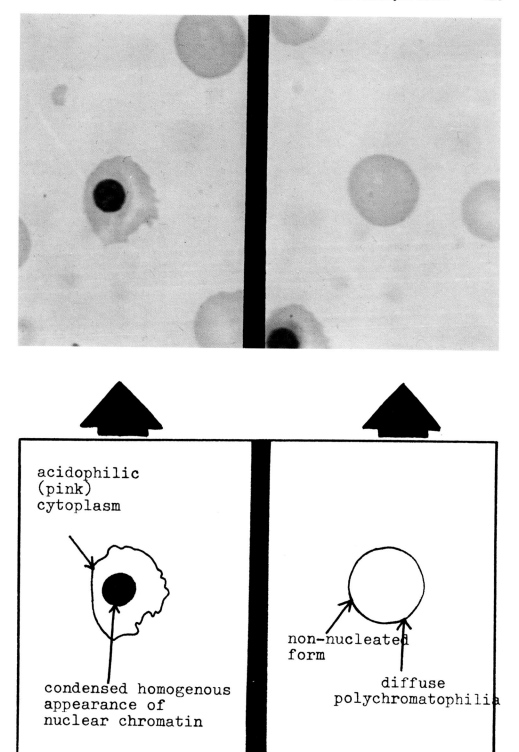

Figure 11.4. *Upper*, metarubricyte *versus* polychromatic erythrocyte. *Lower*, schematic diagram.

Table 11.5
Morphologic Criteria for Rubricytic Series
Key Differentiating Feature:
Change from polychromatophilic to pink cytoplasm and lessening of cell size.

	Polychromatophilic Erythrocyte	Mature Erythrocyte
Cell size	7–10 μm in diameter	6–8 μm in diameter
Nuclear: cytoplasmic ratio (N:C)	—	—
Nuclear shape	—	—
Nuclear position	—	—
Nuclear color and chromatin	—	—
Nucleoli	—	—
Color and amount of cytoplasm	Clear *gray-blue* (*polychromatophilic*) to pink	*Pink*
Cytoplasmic granules	None	None

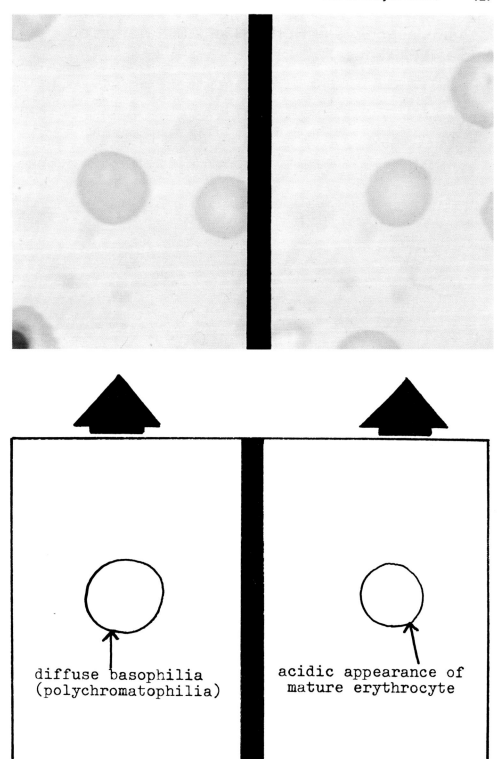

Figure 11.5. *Upper*, polychromatic erythrocyte *versus* mature erythrocyte. *Lower*, schematic diagram.

Megaloblastic *versus* Normoblastic Maturation of Nucleated Stages

The four morphologic characteristics which differentiate megaloblastic maturation from normoblastic maturation are:

1. *Increased parachromatin of megaloblasts* (most important characteristic).
2. *Increased cell size of megaloblasts* (second most important characteristic).
3. *Increased cytoplasm of megaloblsts.*
4. *Asynchronous maturation of megaloblasts*: nuclear maturation lags behind cytoplasmic maturation.

Note: The last two nucleated megaloblastic stages may show a tendency to segmentation or hypersegmentation (see megaloblastic metarubricyte).

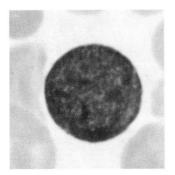

Figure 11.6A.

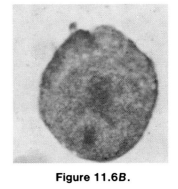

Figure 11.6B.

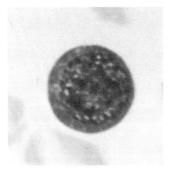

Figure 11.6C.

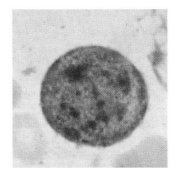

Figure 11.6D.

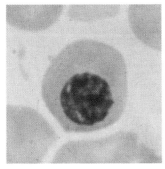

Figure 11.6E.

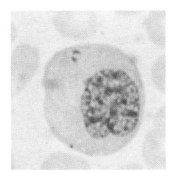

Figure 11.6F.

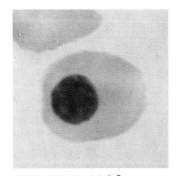

Figure 11.6G.

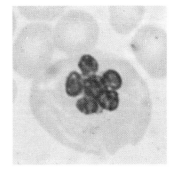

Figure 11.6H.

Figure 11.6. Comparison between normoblastic maturation and megaloblastic maturation (See page 140). *A*, normoblastic rubriblast (original magnification ×1500); *B*, megaloblastic rubriblast (original magnification ×1500); *C*, normoblastic prorubricyte (original magnification ×1500); *D*, megaloblastic prorubricyte (original magnification ×1500); *E*, normoblastic rubricyte (original magnification ×1500); *F*, megaloblastic rubricyte (original magnification ×1500); *G*, normoblastic metarubricyte (original magnification ×1500); *H*, megaloblastic metarubricyte (original magnification ×1500).

Chapter 12

The Reticulocyte

The CAP (College of American Pathologists) Comprehensive Hematology-Clinical Microscopy Survey Program (Series H) of reticulocytes by counts and morphologic identification of reticulocytes from 1971 to 1974 revealed an excessive variance in reticulocyte counts. The survey slides were specifically chosen to illustrate transitional or borderline forms of immature erythrocytes in order to determine more clearly the exact criteria being used for identification throughout the country.[64]

It was discovered that the coefficients of variation (CV) for surveys are 2 to 3 times the levels of intralaboratory variation. This discrepancy appears to be related to a problem with positive reticulocyte identification by the participants. The Survey referee panel results had less variability and could be explained on the basis of a more uniform classification by this group.[64]

It is, therefore, pertinent to review Heilmeyer's[81] classification of reticulocytes which has stood the test of time. Please refer to pages 132 to 134 for photographs and schematic diagrams of his classification of reticulocytes. It is especially important to be aware of Heilmeyer's[81] Group I and IV reticulocyte definitions since these cells gave the most trouble to participants in the CAP survey. The Group I reticulocyte was confused with a normoblast and the Group IV "dotted" reticulocyte is the crux of the controversy. Survey participants appeared to favor the acceptance of a "dotted" reticulocyte. However, in the varied definitions of Group IV reticulocytes, the plural "granules" is used. The consensus of investigations suggests the following minimum criterion for counting a cell as a reticulocyte: a reticulocyte must contain *TWO* or more clumps or discrete blue granules that are visible without requiring fine focus adjustment on the individual cell to confirm their presence. The granules should be away from the cell margin to avoid confusion with Heinz bodies.[64]

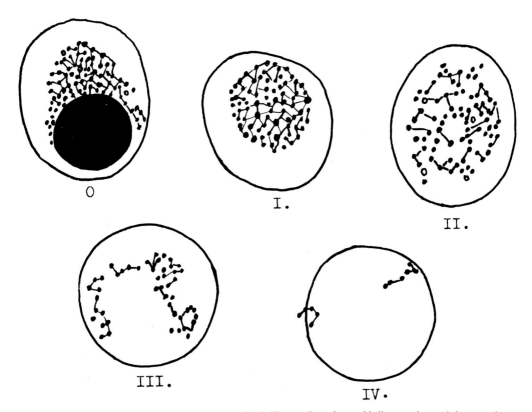

Figure 12.1. Hand drawing of the original illustration from Heilmeyer's article on the morphologic classification of reticulocytes.[81]

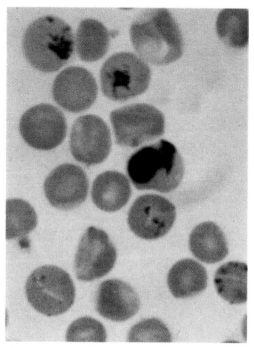

Figure 12.2A. Group O cell (*arrow*) is a normoblast and/or megaloblast that contains both nucleus and a dense perinuclear reticulum. In the cell pictured at left, to which the arrow is pointing, the reticulum is on the upper right of the cell (original magnification ×1500). *DO NOT COUNT AS A RETICULOCYTE!*

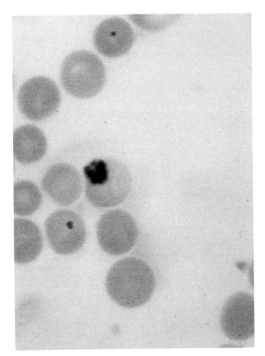

Figure 12.2B. Group I reticulocyte in which reticulum appears in the form of a dense clump.

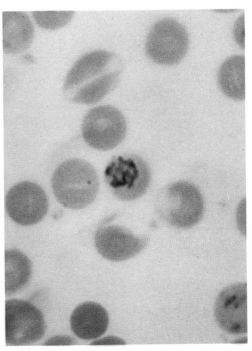

Figure 12.2C. Group II reticulocyte in which reticulum appears in the form of a wreath.

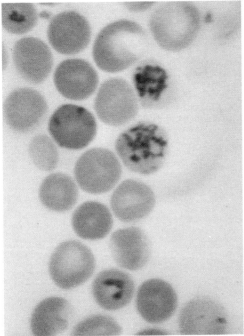

Figure 12.2D. Group III reticulocyte in which the wreath has disintegrated. One-third of circulating reticulocytes.

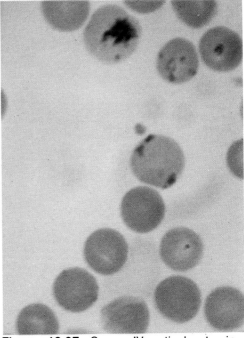

Figure 12.2E. Group IV reticulocyte in which only a few scattered granules of the reticulum remain. Sixty percent of circulating reticulocytes.

Chapter 13

The Comparative Series

Lymphocyte Series *versus* Monocytic Series

Table 13.1
Morphologic Criteria for Comparative Series
Key Differentiating Features:
The nucleus of the smaller prolymphocyte contains clumped blue-purple chromatin with red-purple parachromatin giving a light and dark effect to material and very scanty agranular cytoplasm giving a "bare nucleus" appearance whereas the larger immature monocyte has pale red-purple reticular chromatin and abundant cytoplasm often with fine red granules or particles.

	Immature Lymphocyte	Immature Monocyte
Cell size	9–18 μm in diameter	12–20 μm in diameter
Nuclear: cytoplasmic ratio (N:C)	4:1, occasionally 3:1	3:1 or 2:1
Nuclear shape	Round or indented	Round with chromatin creases or cerebriform folding
Nuclear position	Eccentric with scanty cytoplasm to one side or round	Central
Nuclear color and chromatin	Condensed clumped blue-purple chromatin and red-purple parachromatin (light and dark effect)	Pale red-purple reticular chromatin (aerated network of fine threads)
Nucleoli	0–1	0–2
Color and amount of cytoplasm	Scanty, clear basophilic	Abundant pale gray-basophilia equally proportioned around the nucleus with pseudopodia at border
Cytoplasmic granules	Absent	May or may not contain fine red dust-like particles

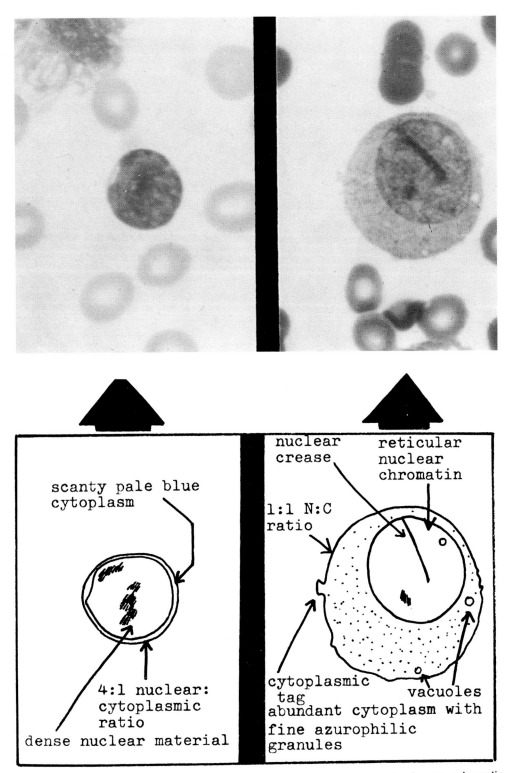

Figure 13.1. *Upper*, immature lymphocyte *versus* immature monocyte. *Lower*, schematic diagram.

Table 13.2
Morphologic Criteria for Comparative Series
Key Differentiating Features:
Mature lymphocyte exhibits dark-staining, dense, homogenous nuclear chromatin with scanty, agranular sky-blue cytoplasm whereas the mature monocyte has pale-staining, fine, reticular nuclear chromatin with abundant, granular, gray-blue cytoplasm.

	Mature Lymphocyte	Mature Monocyte
Cell size	7–18 μm in diameter (most forms 9–12 μm in diameter)	12–20 μm in diameter
Nuclear: cytoplasmic ratio (N:C)	4:1 (occasionally 3:1)	2:1 or 1:1
Nuclear shape	Round or indented	Folded (cerebriform) or narrow, elongated (horseshoe shape)
Nuclear position	Eccentric with scanty cytoplasm to one side or central	Central
Nuclear color and chromatin	Dark-staining, dense homogenous, blue-purple nuclear chromatin pattern	Pale-staining, blue-purple, fine reticular chromatin pattern
Nucleoli	Usually absent rarely one seen in mature form	None
Color and amount of cytoplasm	Light clear sky-blue scanty to moderate	Abundant, pale gray-blue equally proportioned around the nucleus with border pseudopodia, often vacuolated
Cytoplasmic granules	Usually absent, occasionally few azurophilic granules seen	Numerous fine pale red evenly dispersed dust-like particles

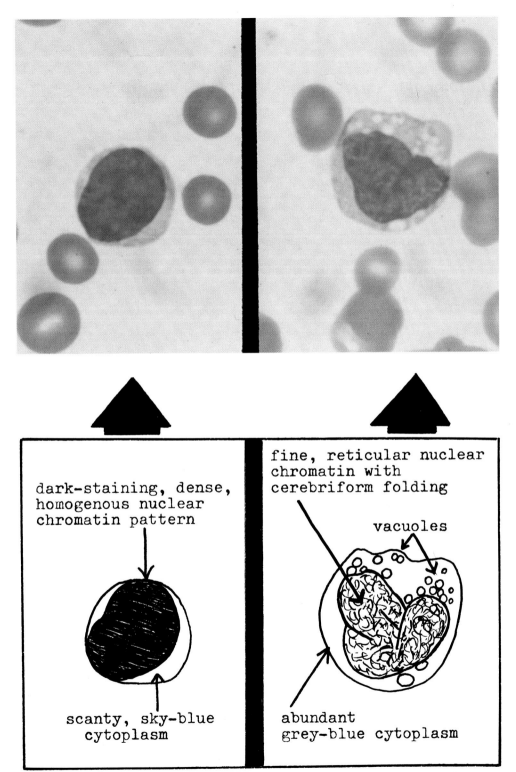

Figure 13.2. *Upper,* mature lymphocyte *versus* mature monocyte. *Lower,* schematic diagram.

Lymphocytic Series *versus* Atypical Lymphocytes

Table 13.3
Morphologic Criteria for Comparative Series
Key Differentiating Features:
The mature lymphocyte is smaller with a uniformly round nucleus with dense blue-purple chromatin and scanty sky-blue cytoplasm (4:1 N:C ratio). The Downey II atypical lymphocyte has an enlarged, irregularly shaped nucleus, frequently with nucleoli, and pale red-purple chromatin with abundant cytoplasm with an irregular scalloping and deeper basophilia at its border.

	Mature Lymphocyte	Downey II Atypical Lymphocyte
Cell size	7–18 μm in diameter	12–20 μm in diameter
Nuclear: cytoplasmic ratio (N:C)	4:1 (occasionally 3:1)	2:1 or 1:1
Nuclear shape	Round or indented	Enlarged, sometimes elongated, clefted, or lobulated
Nuclear position	Eccentric with scanty cytoplasm to one side or round	Usually central, occasionally eccentric
Nuclear color and chromatin	Dark-staining, dense homogenous, blue-purple nuclear chromatin	Moderate staining, homogenous red-purple nuclear chromatin
Nucleoli	Usually absent, rarely one seen	1–4
Color and amount of cytoplasm	Light, clear sky-blue, scanty to moderate	Abundant pale blue with deepest blue at irregular scalloped border with strong tendency to flow round adjacent rbcs
Cytoplasmic granules	Usually absent, occasionally few azurophilic granules seen	Usually absent, occasionally few azurophilic granules seen

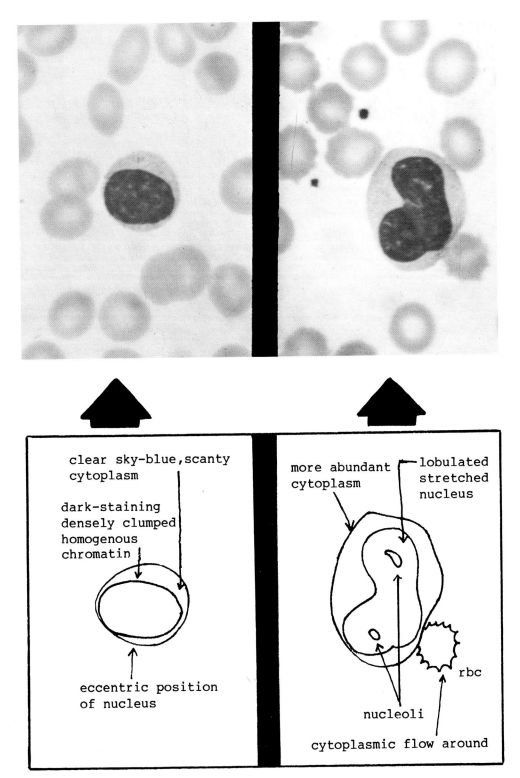

Figure 13.3. *Upper,* mature lymphocyte *versus* Downey Type II atypical lymphocyte. *Lower,* schematic diagram.

Table 13.4
Morphologic Criteria for Comparative Series
Key Differentiating Features:
The Downey III atypical lymphocyte has dense mature nuclear chromatin with abundant cytoplasm (2:1 or 1:1 N:C ratio) which tends to flow round adjacent rbcs whereas immature lymphocytes contain immature nuclear chromatin with scanty cytoplasm (4:1 N:C ratio).

	Downey III Atypical Lymphocyte	Immature Lymphocytes
Cell size	18–32 μm in diameter	9–18 μm in diameter
Nuclear: cytoplasmic ratio (N:C)	2:1 or 1:1	4:1 occasionally 3:1
Nuclear shape	Elongated, irregular	Round or indented
Nuclear position	Usually central	Eccentric with scanty cytoplasm to one side or may be central (bare nucleus effect)
Nuclear color and chromatin	Mature, dense, homogenous, red-purple nuclear chromatin in enlarged nuclear area	Combination of condensed clumped blue-purple chromatin with red-purple parachromatin (light and dark effect)
Nucleoli	1–4	0–1 (less distinct)
Color and amount of cytoplasm	Deeply basophilic, evenly encircles the nucleus, tends to flow round adjacent rbcs	Scanty, clear basophilic
Cytoplasmic granules	Usually absent, rarely azurophilic granules seen	Absent

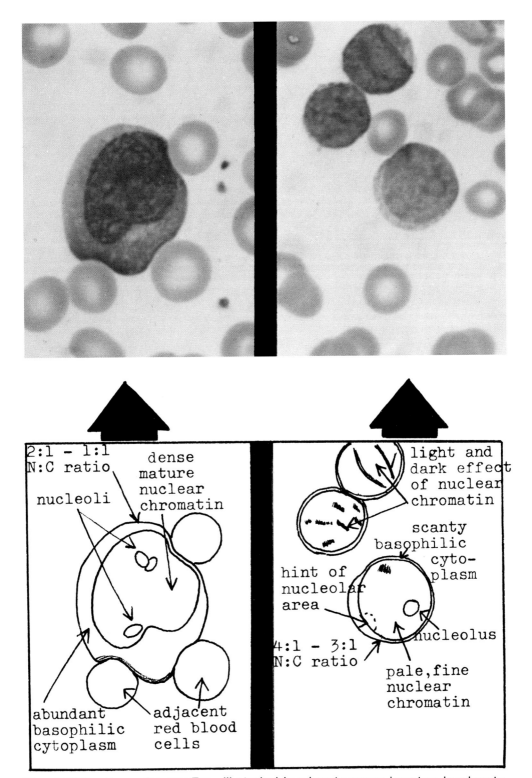

Figure 13.4. *Upper,* Downey Type III atypical lymphocyte *versus* immature lymphocyte. *Lower,* schematic diagram.

Monocytic Series *versus* Myelocytic Series

Table 13.5
Morphologic Criteria for Comparative Series
Key Differentiating Features:
The immature monocyte has a round nucleus with chromatin creases or cerebriform folding with red-purple reticular chromatin and gray-basophilic cytoplasm with border pseudopodia. The cytoplasm is equally proportioned around the nucleus. The promyelocyte has a more eccentric nuclear placement with slightly aggregated chromatin and a one-sided, more basophilic cytoplasm.

	Immature Monocyte	Promyelocyte
Cell size	12–20 μm in diameter	10–20 μm in diameter
Nuclear: cytoplasmic ratio (N:C)	3:1 or 2:1	3:1
Nuclear shape	Round, chromatin creases or cerebriform folding seen	Round or oval
Nuclear position	Central	Eccentric, occasionally central
Nuclear color and chromatin	Pale red-purple reticular chromatin pattern (aerated network of fine threads)	Pale red-purple chromatin with slightly aggregated pattern at nuclear membrane and nucleoli
Nucleoli	0–2	1–5
Color and amount of cytoplasm	Pale gray-basophilic abundant, equally proportioned around the nucleus with pseudopodia at border	Basophilic, tendency to one-sided placement
Cytoplasmic granules	May or may not contain fine red dust-like particles	Present, fine azurophilic, nonspecific granules

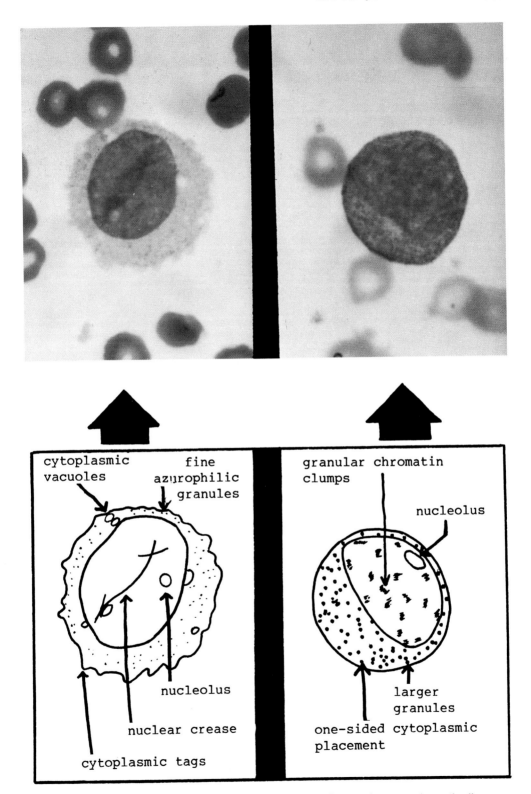

Figure 13.5. *Upper,* immature monocyte *versus* promyelocyte. *Lower,* schematic diagram.

Table 13.6
Morphologic Criteria for Comparative Series
Key Differentiating Features:
The immature monocyte has central folded nucleus often with chromatin creases and fine reticular podia at the border whereas the myelocyte has eccentric rounded or oval nucleus with finely granular chromatin and bluish-pink cytoplasm with smooth border.

	Immature Monocyte	Myelocyte
Cell size	12–20 μm in diameter, large percentage of cells in upper range 18–20 μm	10–18 μm in diameter
Nuclear: cytoplasmic ratio (N:C)	3:1 or 2:1	2:1 or 1:1
Nuclear shape	Cerebriform folding, frequently exhibits chromatin creases	Oval or slightly indented, occasionally round
Nuclear position	Usually central	Commonly eccentric may be central
Nuclear color and chromatin	Pale red-purple reticular pattern (aerated network of threads), very fine	Condensed red-purple fine chromatin with slightly aggregated (granular) pattern
Nucleoli	0–2	May or may not have nucleoli
Color and amount of cytoplasm	Pale gray-basophilia abundant, equally proportioned around nucleus with pseudopodia at border, usually vacuolated	Moderate, bluish-pink
Cytoplasmic granules	May or may not contain fine red dust-like particles	Present, coarse, azurophilic, specific granules, *e.g.*, neutrophilic, etc.

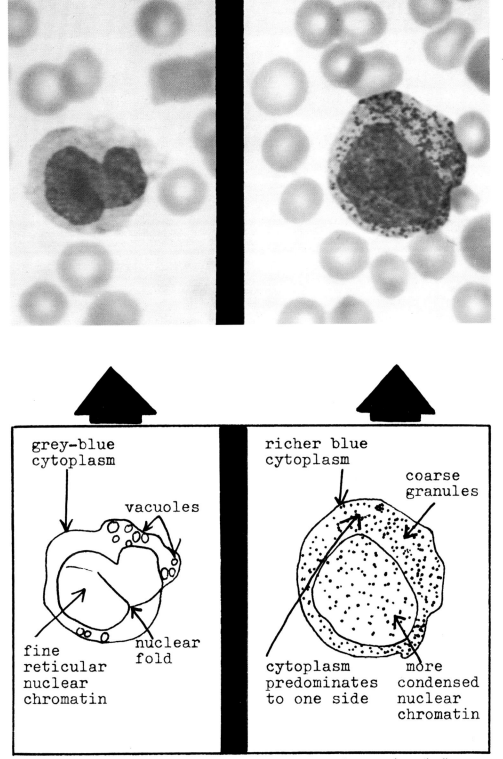

Figure 13.6 *Upper,* immature monocyte *versus* myelocyte. *Lower,* schematic diagram.

Table 13.7
Morphologic Criteria for Comparative Series
Key Differentiating Features:
The nucleus of the segmented monocyte contains fine reticular chromatin and its cytoplasm contains pale red granules throughout whereas the nucleus of the degranulated segmented neutrophil contains coarsely granular chromatin and no or very few granules in its cytoplasm.

	Segmented Monocyte	Degranulated Segmented Neutrophil
Cell size	12–20 μm in diameter	10–16 μm in diameter
Nuclear: cytoplasmic ratio (N:C)	2:1 or 1:1	1:1
Nuclear shape	Cerebriform folding or narrow elongated nucleus (horseshoe shape or segmented)	2–5 distinct nuclear lobes (0.5 μm filament connecting lobes)
Nuclear position	Central	Central or eccentric
Nuclear color and chromatin	Blue-purple fine reticular chromatin	Deep blue-purple coarsely granular chromatin
Nucleoli	None	None
Color and amount of cytoplasm	Gray-blue abundant	Pale blue, abundant
Cytoplasmic granules	Fine pale red dust-like particles evenly dispersed	None or very few specific violet-pink granules

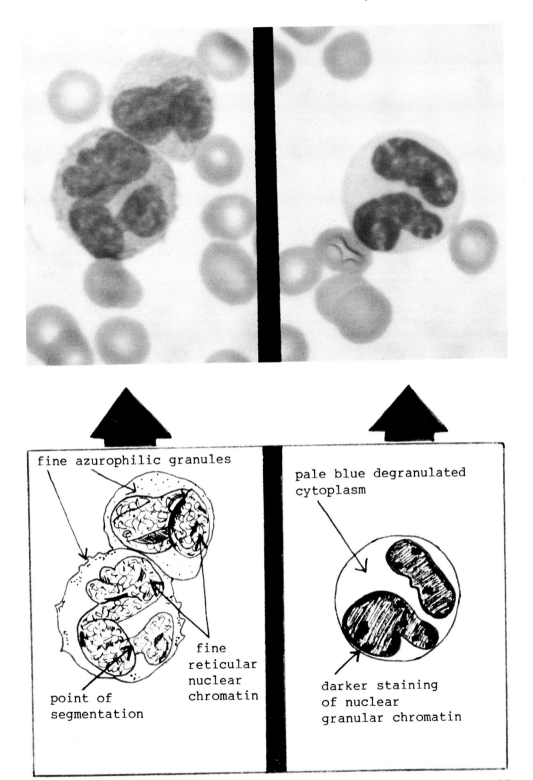

Figure 13.7 *Upper,* segmented monocyte *versus* degranulated segmented neutrophil. *Lower,* schematic diagram.

Table 13.8
Morphologic Criteria for Comparative Series
Key Differentiating Features:
The nucleus of the band neutrophil contains a coarsely granular chromatin pattern and its cytoplasm is clear pink whereas the nucleus of the mature monocyte contains a fine reticular chromatin pattern and its cytoplasm is gray-blue with fine red granules interspersed throughout.

	Band Neutrophil	Mature Monocyte
Cell size	10–16 μm in diameter	12–20 μm in diameter
Nuclear: cytoplasmic ratio (N:C)	1:1	2:1 or 1:1
Nuclear shape	Elongated, narrow band shape of uniform thickness, singular nuclear lobe	Cerebriform folding or narrow elongated nucleus (band shape or horseshoe shape)
Nuclear position	Central or eccentric	Central
Nuclear color and chromatin	Deep blue-purple coarsely granular chromatin	Blue-purple fine reticular chromatin pattern
Nucleoli	None	None
Color and amount of cytoplasm	Abundant pink	Abundant pale gray-blue equally proportioned around nucleus, "bleb-like" pseudopodia at border
Cytoplasmic granules	Specific, fine, violet-pink (lilac)	Fine pale red dust-like particles evenly dispersed

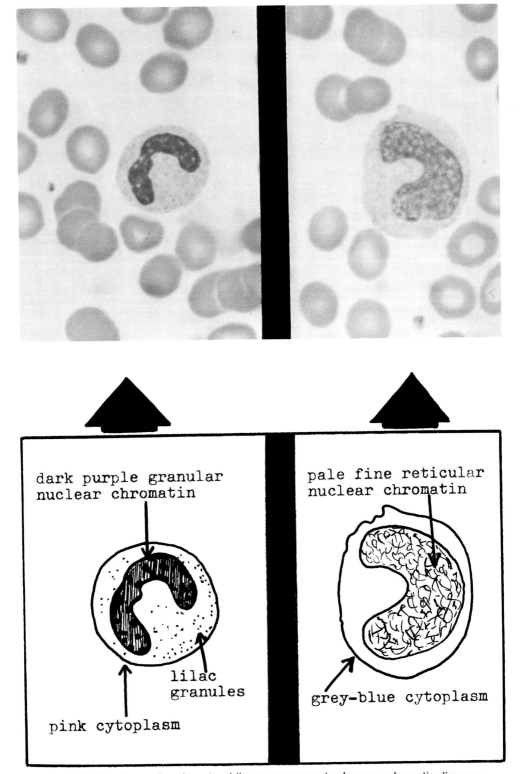

Figure 13.8. *Upper,* band neutrophil *versus* monocyte. *Lower,* schematic diagram.

Plasmacytic Series *versus* Lymphocytic Series

Table 13.9
Morphologic Criteria for Comparative Series
Key Differentiating Features:
The reactive plasmacytoid atypical lymphocyte has an imperfect nuclear shape with predominantly homogenous nuclear chromatin with few isolated dense clumps whereas the mature plasma cell has a perfectly round or oval nuclear shape with persistent granular chromatin clumps throughout the nucleus.

	Reactive Plasmacytoid Atypical (Downey Type I) Lymphocyte	Mature Plasma Cell
Cell size	8–20 µm in diameter	8–20 µm in diameter
Nuclear: cytoplasmic ratio (N:C)	3:1 to 1:1	2:1 or 1:1
Nuclear shape	Usually slightly indented, not uniformly round or oval	Uniformly round or oval
Nuclear position	Frequently eccentric, may be central	Frequently eccentric, occasionally may be central
Nuclear color and chromatin	Predominantly homogenous with isolated dense chromatin clumps (2–3)	Mature blue-purple dense chromatin with large prominent clumps near nuclear margin
Nucleoli	None	None
Color and amount of cytoplasm	One-sided, moderately basophilic, may show vacuoles and perinuclear clear zone	One-sided, moderately basophilic with perinuclear clear zone adjacent to nucleus, often vacuolated
Cytoplasmic granules	Usually none	None

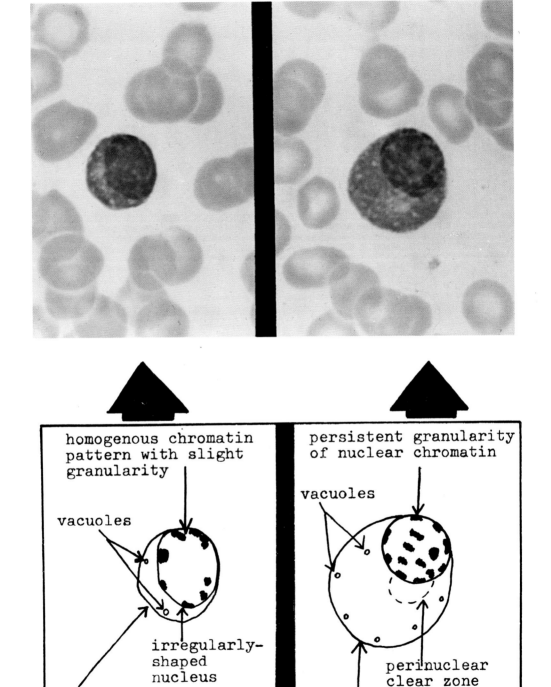

Figure 13.9. *Upper,* Reactive plasmacytoid atypical lymphocyte (RPAL) *versus* mature plasma cell. *Lower,* schematic diagram.

Table 13.10
Morphologic Criteria for Comparative Series
Key Differentiating Features:
The mature plasma cell has an eccentric nucleus (2:1 N:C ratio) with mature blue-purple prominently clumped granular chromatin, adjacent perinuclear clear zone, and one-sided cytoplasm whereas the Downey III atypical lymphocyte has a central nucleus with a red-purple homogenous chromatin and deeply basophilic cytoplasm which encircles the nucleus proportionately with a tendency to flow around adjacent rbcs.

	Mature Plasma Cell	Downey III Atypical Lymphocyte
Cell size	8–20 μm in diameter	18–32 μm in diameter
Nuclear: cytoplasmic ratio (N:C)	2:1 or 1:1	2:1 or 1:1
Nuclear shape	Round or oval	Elongated, irregular
Nuclear position	Frequently eccentric, occasionally may be central	Usually central
Nuclear color and chromatin	Blue-purple dense chromatin with large clumps near nuclear margin (granular pattern)	Dense, homogenous red-purple nuclear chromatin in an enlarged nuclear area
Nucleoli	None	1–4
Color and amount of cytoplasm	Moderate, basophilic with perinuclear clear zone adjacent to nucleus, may contain vacuoles	Deeply basophilic, encircles the nucleus proportionately, tends to flow around adjacent rbcs
Cytoplasmic granules	None	Usually absent, rarely azurophilic granules seen

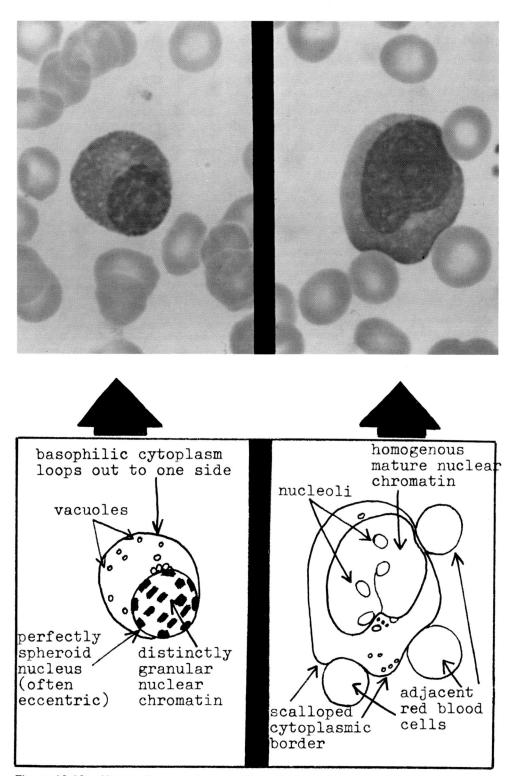

Figure 13.10.   *Upper,* plasma cell *versus* Type III atypical lymphocyte. *Lower,* schematic diagram.

Plasmacytic Series *versus* Rubricytic Series

Table 13.11
Morphologic Criteria for Comparative Series
Key Differentiating Features:
The plasma cell has an eccentric nucleus (2:1 N:C ratio) with *mature* blue-purple prominently clumped granular chromatin, adjacent perinuclear clear zone, and one-sided cytoplasm whereas the rubriblast has a central nucleus (4:1 N:C ratio) with *immature* red-purple, finely stippled nuclear chromatin with cytoplasm circumventing nucleus.

	Mature Plasma Cell	Rubriblast
Cell size	8–20 μm in diameter	14–19 μm in diameter
Nuclear: cytoplasmic ratio (N:C)	*2:1 or 1:1*	*4:1*
Nuclear shape	Round or oval	Round
Nuclear position	*Frequently eccentric,* occasionally may be central	*Central*
Nuclear color and chromatin	*Mature, blue-purple dense chromatin arranged in prominent clumps near nuclear margin*	*Immature, red-purple finely stippled granular chromatin*
Nucleoli	None	0–2
Color and amount of cytoplasm	*One-sided, moderately basophilic with perinuclear clear zone adjacent to nucleus, may contain few vacuoles*	*Intensely* basophilic, *circumvents nucleus*, not vacuolated
Cytoplasmic granules	None	None

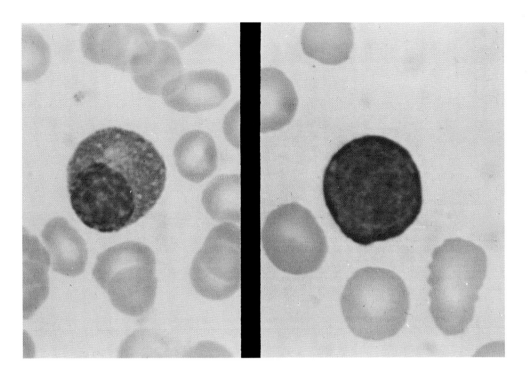

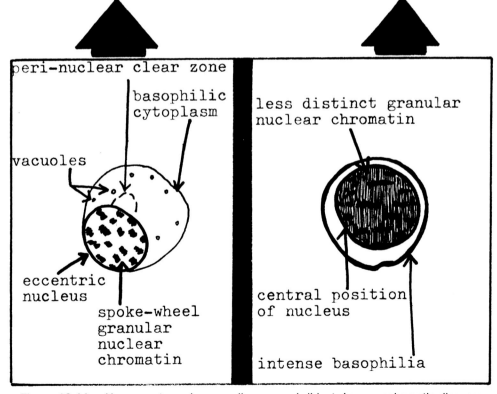

Figure 13.11. *Upper,* mature plasma cell *versus* rubriblast. *Lower,* schematic diagram.

Table 13.12
Morphologic Criteria for Comparative Series
Key Differentiating Features:
Smaller plasma cell has 2:1 or 1:1 N:C ratio, an eccentric nucleus with
mature, prominently clumped chromatin, perinuclear clear zone, and one-
sided cytoplasm whereas the megaloblastic prorubricyte is large (4:1 N:C
ratio), with central nucleus, immature red-purple chromatin with high parachromatin content, cytoplasm circumvents the nucleus and rarely exhibits
a perinuclear clear zone.

	Mature Plasma Cell	Megaloblastic Prorubricyte
Cell size	8–20 μm in diameter	25–35 μm in diameter
Nuclear: cytoplasmic ratio (N:C)	2:1 or 1:1	4:1
Nuclear shape	Round or oval	usually round, rarely oval
Nuclear position	Frequently eccentric, occasionally may be central	Usually central, may be eccentric
Nuclear color and chromatin	Blue-purple, dense, mature chromatin with large promenent clumps near nuclear margin	Red-purple, fine immature chromatin with high parachromatin content
Nucleoli	None	May or may not have nucleoli
Color and amount of cytoplasm	One-sided, moderately basophilic with perinuclear clear zone adjacent to nucleus, may contain vacuoles	Basophilic, evenly arranged around the nucleus, rarely exhibits perinuclear clear zone
Cytoplasmic granules	None	None

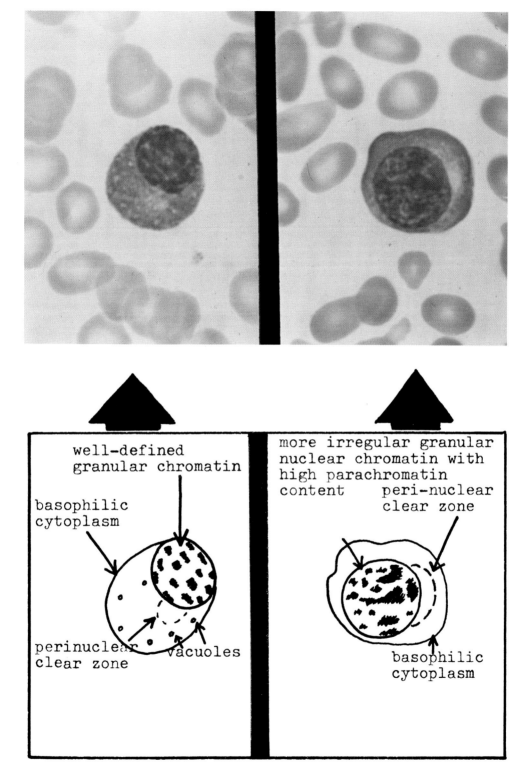

Figure 13.12. *Upper,* mature plasma cell *versus* megaloblastic prorubricyte. *Lower,* schematic diagram.

Neutrophilic Series *versus* Rubricytic Series

Table 13.13
Morphologic Criteria for Comparative Series
Key Differentiating Features:
The hypersegmented neutrophil displays *greater lobulation* of its nucleus
which contains *coarse granular chromatin clumps and clear spaces* with
pink cytoplasm laden with pink-violet granules whereas the hypersegmented rubricyte nucleus contains *immature pale parachromatin and dark
aggregates of chromatin* with *agranular polychromatophilic cytoplasm.*

	Hypersegmented Neutrophil	Hypersegmented Rubricyte
Cell size	10–16 μm in diameter, 15–25 μm in diameter	12–35 μm in diameter, most in 25–35 μm diameter range
Nuclear: cytoplasmic ratio (N:C)	1:1	1:1
Nuclear shape	6–10 or more distinct nuclear lobes (0.5 μm filament connecting lobes)	2–6 or more distinct nuclear lobes
Nuclear position	Central or eccentric	Usually central, may be eccentric
Nuclear color and chromatin	Deep blue-purple coarsely granular chromatin pattern, chromatin aggregation causes clear spaces	Immature pale-staining parachromatin with small dark aggregates of mature chromatin
Nucleoli	None	None
Color and amount of cytoplasm	Abundant, pink	Moderate to abundant, polychromatophilic and opaque, may contain pink areas of hemoglobin near nucleus
Cytoplasmic granules	Specific, fine violet-pink	None

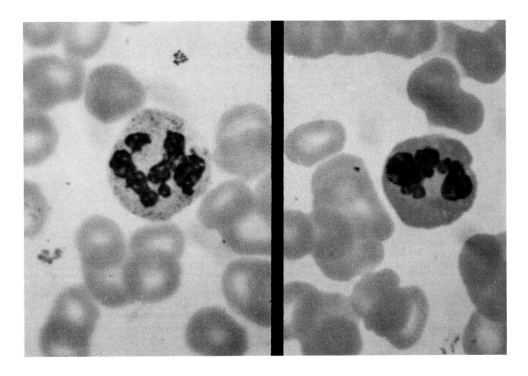

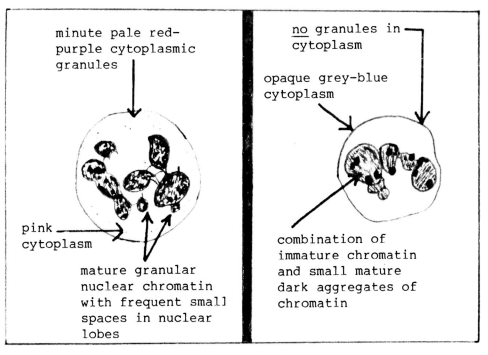

minute pale red-
purple cytoplasmic
granules

<u>no</u> granules in
cytoplasm

opaque grey-blue
cytoplasm

pink
cytoplasm

mature granular
nuclear chromatin
with frequent small
spaces in nuclear
lobes

combination of
immature chromatin
and small mature
dark aggregates of
chromatin

Figure 13.13.   *Upper,* hypersegmented neutrophil *versus* hypersegmented rubricyte (megaloblastic). *Lower,* schematic diagram.

Table 13.14
Morphologic Criteria for Comparative Series
Key Differentiating Features:
The nucleus of the larger metamyelocyte has spaced basi- and oxyphilic granular chromatin and clear pink or bluish-pink cytoplasm containing numerous specific granules whereas the blue-purple nucleus of the smaller metarubricyte displays pyknotic degeneration and condensed chromatin giving it a homogenous appearance and opaque pink or bluish-pink cytoplasm.

	Metamyelocyte	Metarubricyte
Cell size	10–18 μm in diameter	8–12 μm in diameter
Nuclear: cytoplasmic ratio (N:C)	1:1	1:1
Nuclear shape	Usually indented (kidney-shaped), oval and *rarely round*	*Round*
Nuclear position	Central or eccentric	Central
Nuclear color and chromatin	Light blue-purple with spaced basi- and oxyphilic granular chromatin easily distinguishable	Blue-purple small nucleus with pyknotic degeneration and condensed homogenous chromatin
Nucleoli	None	None
Color and amount of cytoplasm	Moderate, clear, usually pink, occasionally bluish-pink	Moderate, opaque, usually pink, occasionally bluish-pink
Cytoplasmic granules	Specific granules, *e.g.*, neutrophilic, etc.	None

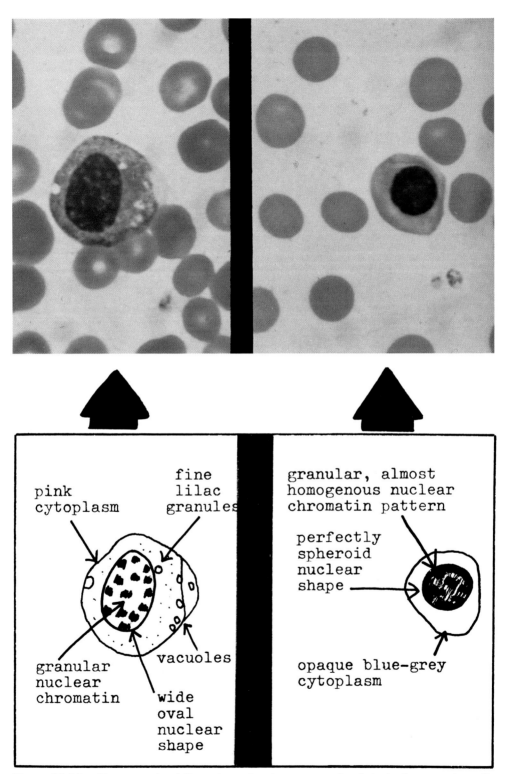

Figure 13.14. *Upper,* neutrophilic metamyelocyte *versus* metarubricyte. *Lower,* schematic diagram.

Miscellaneous Comparisons

Table 13.15
Morphologic Criteria for Comparative Series
Key Differentiating Features:
The leukoblast usually has an irregular nuclear outline with undifferentiated homogenous nuclear chromatin and basophilic cytoplasm with an irregular border whereas the rubriblast usually has a uniformly round nuclear outline with finely stippled granular nuclear chromatin and *intensely* basophilic cytoplasm with a regular border.

	Leukoblast	Rubriblast
Cell size	10–20 μm in diameter	14–19 μm in diameter
Nuclear: cytoplasmic ratio (N:C)	4:1	4:1
Nuclear shape	May be round or oval, *slight indentation more commonly seen in leukemic states*	Round
Nuclear position	Eccentric or central, may be folded in monoblast	Central
Nuclear color and chromatin	*Unidifferentiated* pale *homogenous* purple nuclear chromatin	Red-purple *finely stippled granular chromatin*
Nucleoli	1–5	0–2
Color and amount of cytoplasm	Basophilic and scanty, irregular border frequently	*Intensely* basophilic, consistently regular border
Cytoplasmic granules	None	None

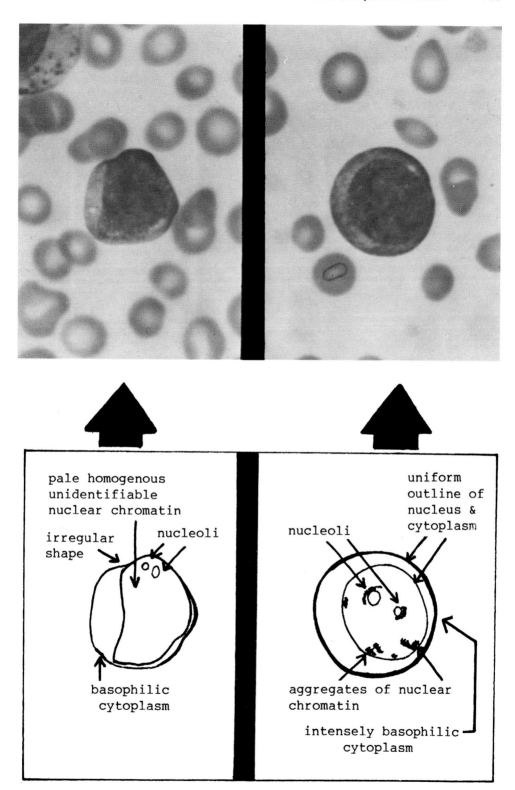

Figure 13.15. *Upper,* leukoblast *versus* rubriblast. *Lower,* schematic diagram.

DEGENERATIVE NUCLEAR FORMS: THE BASKET FORM VERSUS THE SMUDGE FORM

"Basket cell" and "smudge form" are terms used to describe degenerative nuclear remnants occasionally seen in peripheral blood smears.

A *"basket cell"* is a reddish-purple nuclear remnant having *a widely spaced thready network appearance with a more condensed central portion* which may exhibit a nucleolar remnant. The nuclear material appears liquefied and devoid of chromatin pattern. There is no evidence of a cytoplasmic membrane. Monocytes which are large cells with folded nuclei and a loosely spaced nuclear chromatin are examples of cells that commonly demonstrate "basket cell" formation upon degeneration.

A *"smudge form"* is a reddish-purple nuclear remnant with a *compact arrangement of material* occasionally exhibiting one or two indistinct nucleolar areas. The nuclear material appears liquefied and is devoid of chromatin pattern. There is no evidence of a cytoplasmic membrane. Smaller cells with round nuclei and dense chromatin such as a lymphocyte or a nucleated rbc tend to form "smudge forms" upon degeneration.

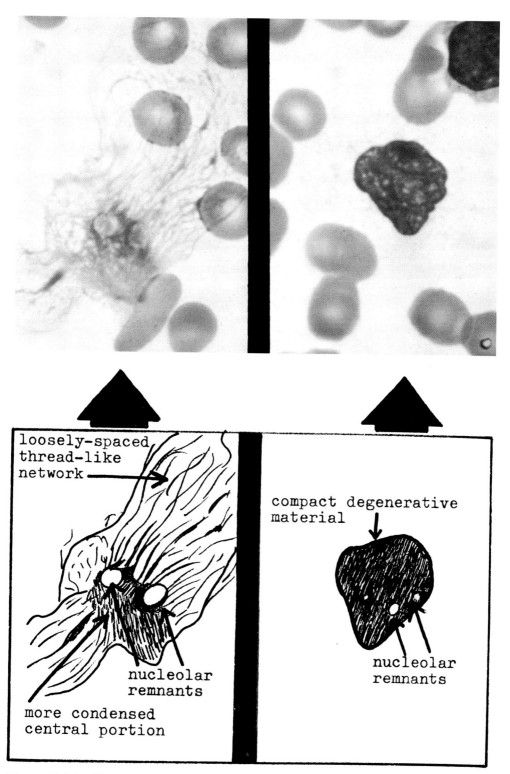

Figure 13.16. *Upper,* degenerative nuclear forms: the basket form *versus* the smudge form. *Lower,* schematic diagram.

Table 13.16
Morphologic Criteria for Comparative Series
Key Differentiating Features:
The platelet has a light blue cytoplasmic membrane (the hyalomere) with evenly dispersed red-purple granules (the chromomere or granulomere) whereas the polychromatophilic erythrocyte has agranular, opaque, gray-blue cytoplasm.

	Platelet	Polychromatophilic Erythrocyte
Cell size	2–4 μm in diameter, giant forms 5–20 μm in diameter	7–10 μm in diameter
Nuclear: cytoplasmic ratio (N:C)	Not applicable, no nucleus	Not applicable, no nucleus
Nuclear shape	—	—
Nuclear position	—	—
Nuclear color and chromatin	—	—
Nucleoli	—	—
Color and amount of cytoplasm	Light blue (hyalomere)	Clear gray-blue (polychromatophilic) to pink
Cytoplasmic granules	Evenly dispersed fine red-purple granules (chromomere or granulomere)	None

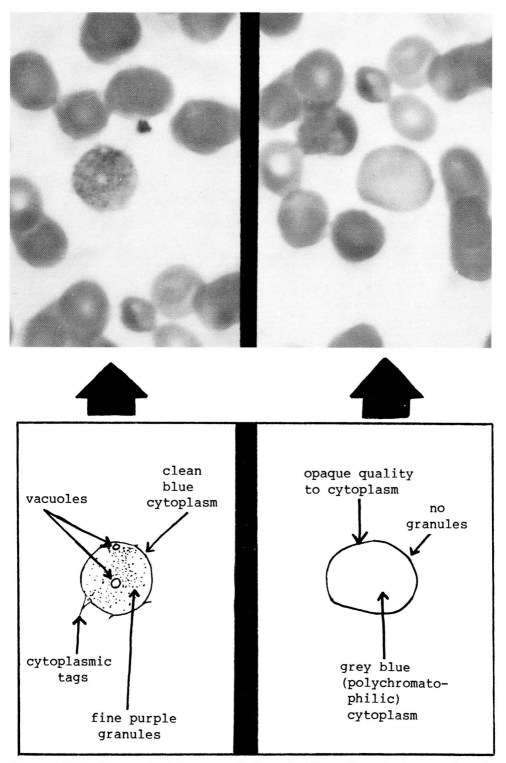

Figure 13.17.   *Upper,* platelet *versus* polychromatophilic erythrocyte. *Lower,* schematic diagram.

Table 13.17
Morphologic Criteria for Comparative Series
Key Differentiating Features:
The smaller myelocyte has a persistent finely granular chromatin throughout the nucleus with loosely spaced coarse specific cytoplasmic granules
with a smooth border whereas the promegakaryocyte has isolated denser
chromatin clumps amid finer immature chromatin with closely spaced
cytoplasmic granules with pseudopodia at the border frequently.

	Myelocyte	Promegakaryocyte
Cell size	10–18 μm in diameter	20–80 μm in diameter
Nuclear: cytoplasmic ratio (N:C)	2:1 or 1:1	4:1–1:1
Nuclear shape	Oval or slightly indented, occasionally round	Usually single, round, oval, indented, or kidney-shaped (rarely multinucleated forms)
Nuclear position	Commonly eccentric, may be central	Central or eccentric
Nuclear color and chromatin	Condensed red-purple fine chromatin with slightly aggregated (granular) pattern throughout nucleus	1–4 smudged, dense chromatin clumps amid fine red-purple immature chromatin
Nucleoli	May or may not have nucleoli	1–5
Color and amount of cytoplasm	Moderate, bluish-pink	Usually abundant with pseudopidia basophilic but paler as maturity approaches
Cytoplasmic granules	Loosely spaced coarse azurophilic, specific granules, e.g., neutrophilic, etc.	Closely spaced fine azurophilic, granules most abundant adjacent to nucleus

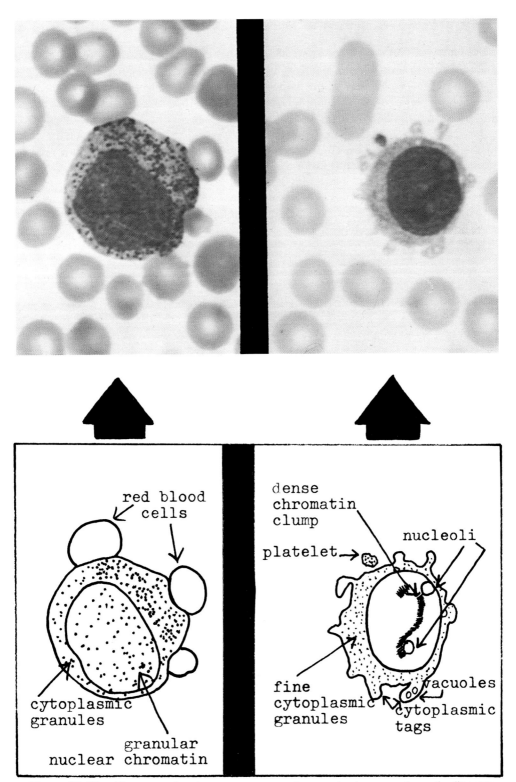

Figure 13.18. *Upper,* myelocyte *versus* promegakaryocyte. *Lower,* schematic diagram.

Segmental Neutrophils *versus* Band Neutrophils

The differentiation between band neutrophils and segmented neutrophils is based upon an astute observation of the marginations and shape of the nucleus. If one judges that the nucleus is one continuous body or lobe with the entire nuclear area showing chromatin pattern between the borders, then it is identified as a nonsegmented neutrophil or band form. Some hematologists use a third synonym for this cell, "stab form." However, if one sees that the nucleus appears to be two lobes or more connected by fine filaments or threads usually less than 1 μm in diameter[57] and showing no nuclear chromatin between borders at these points then one must identify this cell as a segmented neutrophil or polymorphonuclear leukocyte. The decision is not always this clear-cut, unfortunately. Some cells do not show fine filaments connecting the nuclear lobes, but we can tell by the margins and indentations that the nucleus is most likely segmented but the filament is either hidden or broken. The following schematic diagrams are illustrative of this point:

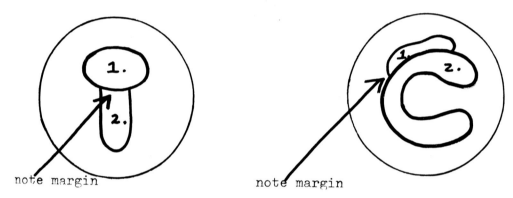

note margin   note margin

In these instances I instruct my students to carefully outline the shape of the nucleus with their eyes and if they find that in so doing they close all borders completely on one given section of the nucleus without crossing a margination or line, and there is still excess nucleus then it is two lobes or more and is identified as a segmented neutrophil.

However, if in outlining the nucleus, they include and close all borders of as one section, and there is no excess nucleus then it is identified as a nonsegmented neutrophil. The following schematic diagrams depict the visual outlining with a dotted line:

In borderline decisions where the differentiation is extremely difficult, it is wise to give the cell the benefit of the doubt, so to speak, and identify it as the more mature form, the segmented neutrophil.

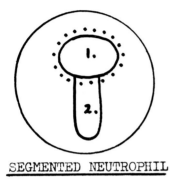

SEGMENTED NEUTROPHIL

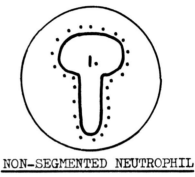

NON-SEGMENTED NEUTROPHIL

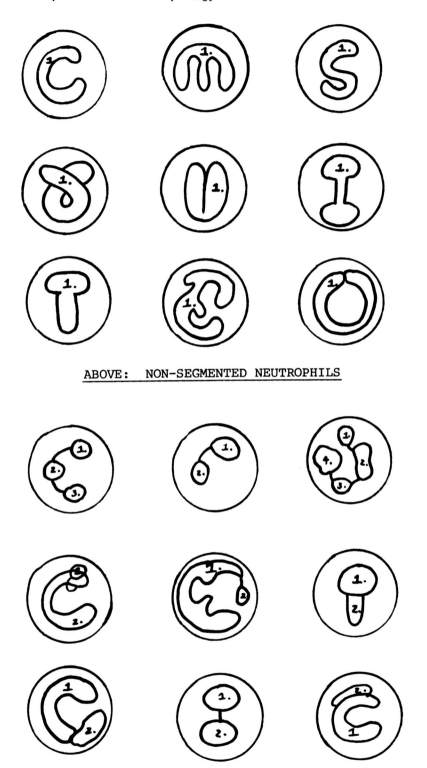

ABOVE: NON–SEGMENTED NEUTROPHILS

ABOVE: SEGMENTED NEUTROPHILS

Figure 13.19.   Nonsegmented neutrophils (*upper*) versus segmented neutrophils (*lower*)

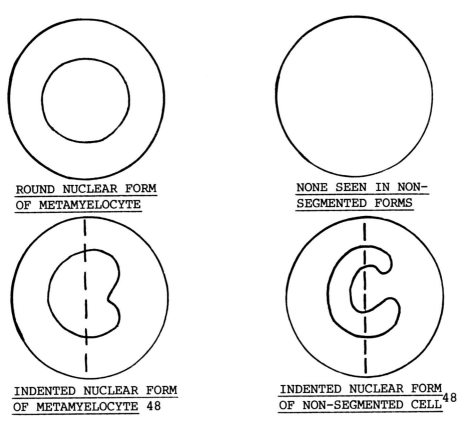

ROUND NUCLEAR FORM
OF METAMYELOCYTE

NONE SEEN IN NON-
SEGMENTED FORMS

INDENTED NUCLEAR FORM
OF METAMYELOCYTE 48

INDENTED NUCLEAR FORM
OF NON-SEGMENTED CELL[48]

The differentiation is based on degree of nuclear indentation. Imagine a mid-nuclear line and if the indentation remains before the mid-nuclear line, the nucleus is wide enough to be identified as a metamyelocyte. If the indentation extends beyond the mid-nuclear line, then the nucleus has narrowed and elongated sufficiently to be identified as a non-segmented neutrophil.[48]

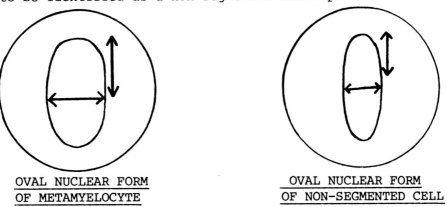

OVAL NUCLEAR FORM
OF METAMYELOCYTE

OVAL NUCLEAR FORM
OF NON-SEGMENTED CELL

In this type of nucleus, look at the width of the nucleus and then imagine you could transpose it to the length of the nucleus. If the width is half the length of the nucleus, identify as metamyelocyte; if the width is less than half the length, identify as non-segmented form.

Figure 13.20. Metamyelocytes *versus* band neutrophils.

Chapter 14

Morphology of Erythrocytes in Disease

Definition of the Mature Erythrocyte (Normocyte)

Hypochromia. The normal erythrocyte does not exhibit true hypochromia but may show slight central pallor not exceeding one-third the diameter of the cell.

Anisocytosis. The normal erythrocyte is 6–8 μm in diameter with an average of 7.2 μm, a thickness of 2 μm, and a volume of 90 μm^3.[31,85]

Poikilocytosis. The normal erythrocyte is a biconcave disc on cross-section and a round globule on top view as seen on Wright-stained smears.[31]

Polychromasia. The normal erythrocyte population contains 0.5–2% cells with a diffuse pale gray-blue hue due to ribosomal protein which is indicative of immaturity.

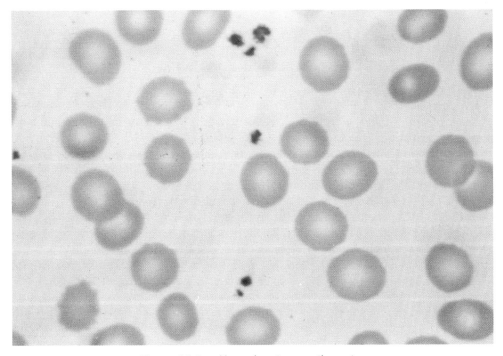

Figure 14.1. Normal mature erythrocytes.

The Macrocytic Anemias

B₁₂-FOLATE DEFICIENCY ANEMIAS

Key Words: Macrocytic Ovalocytosis, Hypersegmentation

B$_{12}$ or folate deficiency anemias cannot be differentiated on a peripheral blood smear. Increased mean corpuscular volume MCV) is usually the first indication in a hematology laboratory doing a Coulter S profile on the blood of a patient to suspect either: 1) B$_{12}$ or folate deficiency, 2) obstructive liver disease, or 3) a combination of both. The MCV is usually between 110–120 fl in most patients and may go as high as 140 fl in severe cases.[76,104] The two principal findings on the peripheral blood smear are hypersegmentation of the granulocytes and a macroovalocytosis of the erythrocytes. The granulocytes should be carefully scrutinized and, if more than three five-lobed polymorphonuclear leukocyte or any polymorphonuclear leukocyte with six lobes or more are seen in the 100-cell differential scan, they should be reported on the patient's requisition.[187] The oval macrocytes are well filled with hemoglobin and tend to predominate but there may be great variability in size with a moderate number of microcytes due to the increased ineffective erythropoiesis seen in these deficiencies. Marked poikilocytosis consisting of teardrops, dumbbells, etc., may be seen in severe anemia. Megaloblastic nucleated rbcs may be present in the peripheral blood of these patients as well as normoblastic nucleated rbcs. To enhance the finding of megaloblastic rbc precursors in peripheral blood smears, 1 cc of the blood sample can be centrifuged to make buffy coat smears and these can then be examined for megaloblastic rbc precursors to increase morphologic evidence for B$_{12}$ or folate deficiency. There may be leukopenia and thrombocytopenia in untreated advanced cases. Some platelets are large and bizarre in shape, especially in B$_{12}$ deficiency.

ANEMIA OF LIVER DISEASE

Key Words: Macrocytosis, Target Cells

Despite the considerable diversity in the etiologic processes (infectious, toxic, degenerative, deficiency) that may be responsible for chronic liver disease, the associated anemias present similar morphologic characteristics. Several types of anemia may coexist with hepatic disease so one must recognize the hematologic changes characteristic of lack of iron, hemoglobinopathy, hereditary or acquired hemolytic disease, B$_{12}$ or folate deficiency, bone marrow failure, etc., and the modification of these by the superimposed changes of the anemia of liver disease.[76] The anemia is usually moderate in degree and rarely severe. The red cells may be mildly macrocytic (MCV 100–115 fl) One study of 222 patients with liver disease showed a high MCV in 137 (62%).[19] The red cells, however, may be normochromic, normocytic in uncomplicated cases. Macrocytosis is most commonly seen in obstructive liver disease. The major poikilocyte is the target cell or leptocyte. The variation in size and shapes is not as extreme as in B$_{12}$ or folate deficiency. Numerous studies have demonstrated a decreased red blood cell survival, so a definite hemolytic process is present and contributing to the anemia. It is wise to make a scan for spherocytes in patients with chronic liver disease, since they are seen in a large proportion of cases. The spherocytes are usually few in number and might be missed unless one makes a concerted effort to find them on peripheral smears. Leukocyte abnormalities have been observed. Some patients have lymphopenia, some

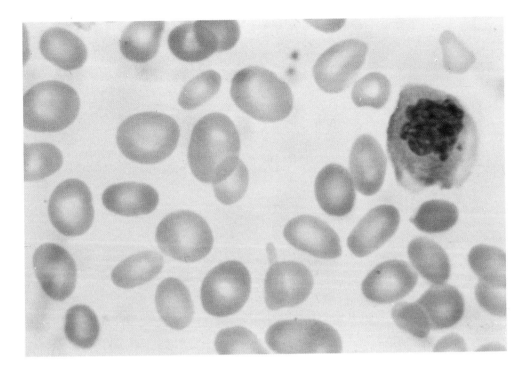

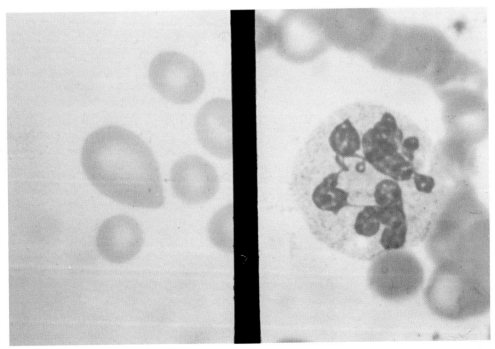

Figure 14.2.   *Top*, B$_{12}$-folate deficiency (original magnification ×1050). Note megaloblastic rubricyte and oval macrocytosis. *Bottom*, megalocyte and hypersegmented neutrophil in B$_{12}$-folate deficiency.

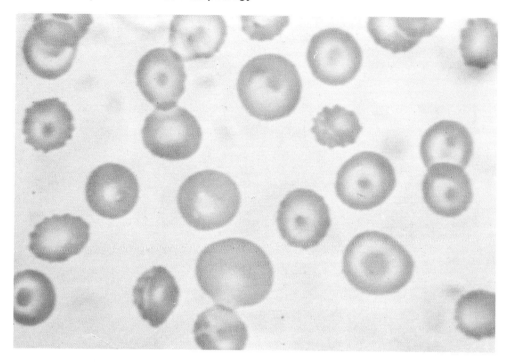

Figure 14.3.   Obstructive liver disease (original magnification ×1500). Note macrocytes and target cells.

have neutropenia, and still others have shown neutrophilia. Mild thrombocytopenia is found in approximately 50% of patients with cirrhosis of the liver.[16,160,187]

Reticulocytes are often increased with counts from 2.3–24.6% resulting in a mean of 8.6%.[187] The reticulocytosis can be suppressed by alcohol ingestion. Therefore, if alcohol intake has continued until the patient is first seen, the reticulocyte count will be low. Upon withdrawal of alcohol, the reticulocytes will increase reaching a maximal level in 7 days.

Red cell precursors in the bone marrow have been described as "macronormoblasts" which implies increased cell size with a normal nuclear chromatin structure. In 20% of patients, however, a frank megaloblastosis may be seen.[16]

The Normocytic Anemias

THE DIFFERENTIATION OF HEMOLYTIC ANEMIAS

In patients who are seen with the usual manifestations of a hemolytic process, such as shortened red cell survival time, elevated serum bilirubin, increased fecal urobilinogen excretion, anemia, reticulocytosis, and splenomegaly, the etiology of their hemolysis has to be determined.[104] The best test to run first is the Coombs test to establish whether or not the hemolysis is due to the presence of antibodies on the rbc surface. If the result of the Coombs test is positive, one must consider autoimmune hemolytic anemia or isoimmune hemolytic disease, such as erythroblastosis fetalis or incompatible blood transfusion. If the result of the Coombs test is negative, one must determine whether the problem is intracorpuscular or extracorpuscular. Extracorpuscular causes of hemolytic anemia are hypersplenism, or mechanical causes, such as a defective prosthetic heart valve, March hemoglobinuria, burns, or metastatic cancer. The possibility of disseminated intravascular coagulation should also be evaluated. Intracorpuscular causes of hemolytic anemia could be subdivided by performing an osmotic fragility test. If there is increased fragility, one would suspect hereditary spherocytosis, hereditary elliptocytosis with hemolysis, etc. If results of fragility tests are normal or decreased fragility, hemoglobin electrophoresis should be performed to detect the presence of an abnormal hemoglobin as the cause of the hemolysis, as found in sickle cell anemia, thalassemia, or hemoglobin C disease. If the result of the hemoglobin electrophoresis is normal, the possibility of a rbc enzyme deficiency (a nonspherocytic hemolytic anemia), such as glucose 6-phosphodiesterase deficiency or pyruvate kinase deficiency, must be investigated. Also tests for paroxysmal nocturnal hemoglobinuria and unstable hemoglobins, which are not detected by electrophoresis, should be performed.

ACQUIRED AUTOIMMUNE HEMOLYTIC ANEMIA

Autoimmune hemolytic anemia (AIHA) is usually divided into two types: 1) primary or idiopathic when no other disease is demonstrable or 2) secondary or symptomatic when associated with some other disease. Three hypotheses have been proposed in an attempt to explain why a patient develops autoantibodies against his own rbcs: 1) alteration of rbc antigen by viruses, bacteria, or drugs such as methyldopa so that the rbcs become antigenic for normal lymphoid cells, 2) cross-reaction with an rbc antigen, and 3) induction of lymphoid cells to produce antibodies against normal rbcs.[104] Since most secondary immune hemolytic anemias are associated with lymphoproliferative disorders, investigators theorize that a mutant clone of lymphocytes may make antibodies against normal lymphocytes. Antibodies in AIHA may be classified according to whether they react optimally at 37°C (warm antibodies (IgG)) or at 4°C (cold antibodies (IgM)).[104]

Warm (IgG)
Idiopathic
Secondary
   Drugs (methyldopa, etc.)
   Lymphoproliferative disorders
   Systemic lupus erythematosus and other
     collagen diseases
   Infections

Cold (IgM)
Idiopathic: cold aggregation
Secondary
   Lymphoproliferative disorders
   Systemic lupus erythematosus and other
     collagen diseases
   Infections
   Paroxysmal nocturnal hemoglobinuria

In AIHA the MCV may be normal but is usually increased (>94 fl) due to the regenerative polychromatophilia macrocytosis (reticulocytosis). There may be anywhere from only an occasional spherocyte to marked numbers of microspherocytes on peripheral blood smears. Schistocytes, acanthocytes, and burr cells may also be seen. Nucleated rbcs are commonly found as well as occasional Howell-Jolly bodies. Erythrophagocytosis by monocytes is sometimes evident in routine smears and may suggest the diagnosis.[183,189] Autoagglutination due to cold agglutinins may be observed and is distinguished from rouleaux formation by its disappearance upon warming the blood or the addition of saline to the blood.[104] Leukocytosis is present during periods of active hemolysis and the increase primarily involves the myelogenous series with myelocytes evident on the peripheral blood smear. Platelet counts are usually normal or moderately

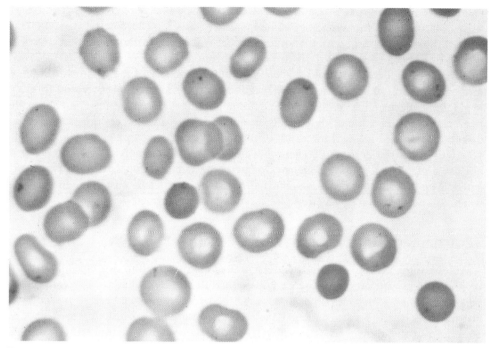

Figure 14.4.   Acquired autoimmune hemolytic anemia. Note two spherocytes exhibiting deeper red-orange color (original magnification ×1050).

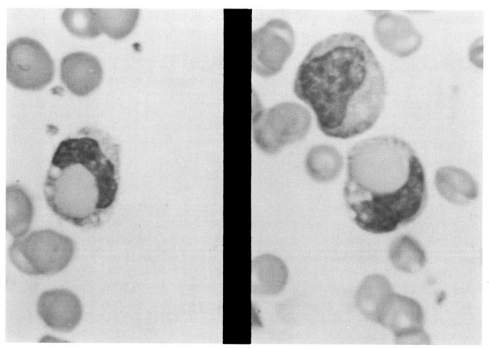

Figure 14.5.   Erythrophagocytosis.

reduced and rarely severely reduced. These peripheral blood findings would warrant the performance of a direct Coombs test to demonstrate the presence of rbc antibodies and confirm the autoimmune nature of the disorder.

ERYTHROPHAGOCYTOSIS

Erythrophagocytosis is the term used to describe the ingestion of whole red blood cells by monocytes most commonly, neutrophils, or by fixed macrophages of the reticuloendothelial system.[187] It is uncommonly seen on routine peripheral blood smears or on buffy coat smears. It is suggestive of damage to the red cell surface, especially that induced by complement-fixing antibodies, but also by protozoan and bacterial infectious agents and certain chemical poisons.[157,170] It is often assumed that erythrophagocytosis is an important mechanism for the disposal of normal, senescent red blood cells, but there is very little direct evidence for this assumption.[189] Erythrophagocytosis is primarily a pathologic phenomenon most commonly observed in autoimmune hemolytic anemia.

MICROANGIOPATHIC HEMOLYTIC ANEMIA (MAHA)

The term "microangiopathic hemolytic anemia" was used in 1962 by Brain et al[27] to describe hemolytic anemia occurring in a variety of disorders which have in common disease of the small blood vessels resulting in partial obstruction of the microvasculature to the flow of erythrocytes. These investigators realized the similarity between the blood smears in these patients and those previously described in patients with traumatic hemolysis secondary to valvular heart disease. In both instances burr cells, schistocytes, and spherocytes were noted. They postulated that the mechanism of hemolysis was trauma to rbcs by turbulent flow across abnormal valves in one and squeezing through virtually obstructed and abnormal small blood vessels in the other.[104]

The following disorders are associated with microangiopathic hemolytic anemia:

Carcinomatosis involving small blood vessels
Thrombotic thrombocytopenia purpura
Disseminated intravascular coagulation
Hemolytic-uremic syndrome of childhood
Malignant hypertension
Acute glomerulonephritis
Lupus erythematosus
Rejection of renal homografts
Purpura fulminans
Eclampsia
Scleroderma
Amyloidosis
Renal cortical necrosis
Polyarteritis
Hemangiomas

MAHA has been induced experimentally in animals by: 1) inducing the generalized Shwartzman reaction[25–27]; 2) injecting thrombin; 3) causing defibrination by injecting purified coagulant fraction of Malayan pit-viper venom[104,152]; and 4) producing malignant hypertension by giving salt overload and desoxycorticosterone.[175]

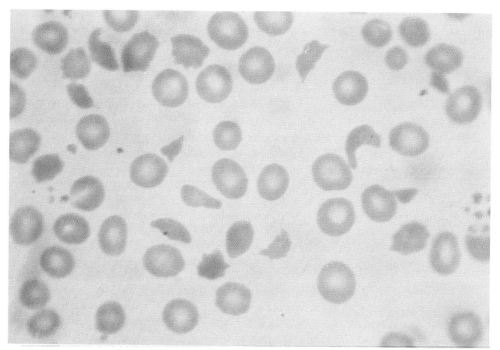

Figure 14.6.   Microangiopathic hemolytic anemia (original magnification ×600).

In these experiments, rbcs were seen enmeshed in fibrin clots, adhered to fibrin on vessel walls, and adhered to damaged endothelium. This rbc adherence plus the force of blood flow through partially occluded small vessels leads to shear stresses causing rbc fragmentation and traumatic hemolysis.[29] The morphologist should carefully scrutinize peripheral blood smears in patients with anemia so the characteristic finding of fragmented rbcs and burr cells is not missed. This finding may provide the first clue to the physician to the nature of the pathologic mechanism of the anemia and the underlying disease.[104]

ERYTHROBLASTOSIS FETALIS (HEMOLYTIC DISEASE OF THE NEWBORN)

Erythroblastosis fetalis is a hemolytic anemia which results when fetal red cells, possessing an antigen which is absent in the mother, cross the placenta into the maternal circulation, where they stimulate production of antibodies. These antibodies then return to the fetal circulation and attach to the antigenic site on the rbc surface leading to destruction of the cell. This hemolytic process takes place *in utero* and results in a marked compensatory overproduction of young nucleated red cells in the fetal erythropoietic sites—thus, the term erythroblastosis fetalis.[187] Allen and Diamond[2] state that ABO incompatibility is responsible for approximately two-thirds of the cases of erythroblastosis fetalis. Rh (D) incompatibility is responsible for about one-third of the cases and other blood factors (c, E, E^w, and Kell) for 2–3%. However, Rh incompatibility causes the greater clinical severity.

Anemia, reticulocytosis, and nucleated rbcs are the major findings in the peripheral blood. Determination of hemoglobin in cord venous blood most accurately indicates the severity of the hemolytic process. Anemia is considered to be present if the hemoglobin level of the cord blood is less than 14 g/100 ml, if the hemoglobin level of the venous blood is less than 15 g/100 ml, or if the hemoglobin level of capillary blood is less than 16 g/100 ml on the first day.[127,131] A hemoglobin level of less than 9 g/100

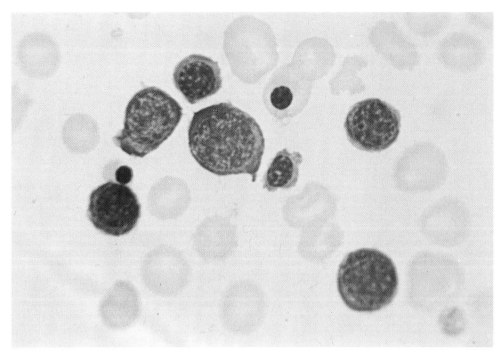

Figure 14.7.   Erythroblastosis fetalis (hemolytic disease of the newborn) (original magnification ×1050).

ml at birth indicates severe anemia. Reticulocytosis is usually greater than 6%[131] and may be as high as 60%.[187] All stages of nucleated rbcs are present in the peripheral blood but the late stages are the more common finding. The nucleated rbcs are very large, but they are not megaloblastic as originally thought.[146] Spherocytosis is characteristic of ABO incompatibility but is usually not seen in Rh incompatibility.[104] Polychromatophilia is marked. The rbcs are usually macrocytic and well filled with hemoglobin. Measurements of red blood cell diameter show a biphasic curve with a macrocytic and a normocytic peak or two macrocytic peaks.[146] Leukocytosis is usually present with the increase mainly in the neutrophilic series. Platelet counts are usually normal, but thrombocytopenia often occurs in the severe cases.[187]

ANEMIA DUE TO SEVERE THERMAL BURNS

The anemia due to severe thermal burns is characteristically hemolytic with hemoglobinemia and hemoglobinuria.[73] The peripheral blood smear shows many microspherocytes, red blood cell fragmentation, and budding.[104] These spherocytes and fragments lack deformability and are sequestered prematurely in the spleen.[76] These patients demonstrate an increased osmotic fragility.

Similar alterations in red blood cell morphology and osmotic fragility can be produced by heating blood a few minutes *in vitro* to temperatures between 47–50°C which causes membrane damage leading to red blood cell sphering and decreased survival. The degree of the anemia is related to the surface area of the body involved and the severity of the burn.[104]

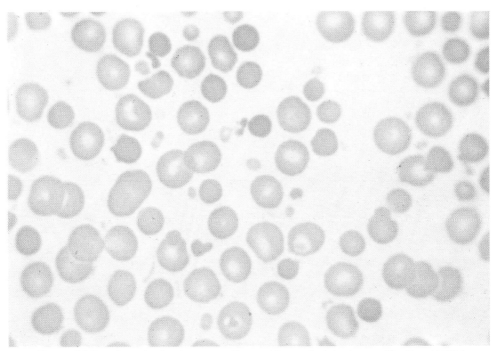

Figure 14.8.   Anemia due to severe thermal burns (original magnification ×600).

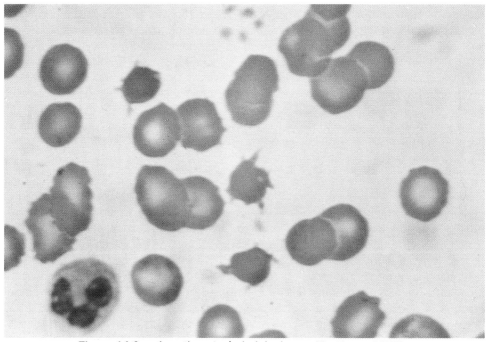

Figure 14.9.   Acanthocytosis (original magnification ×1050).

ACANTHOCYTOSIS (THORN-LIKE PROJECTIONS, SPUR CELLS)

The acanthocyte (spur cell) may be defined as a mature erythrocyte which usually displays 2–10 spicules of varying length and irregular arrangement resembling a spherocyte with pseudopods.[184] Acanthocytes were described by Bassen and Kornzweig in a young girl with a rare syndrome consisting of atypical retinitis pigmentosa, steatorrhea, ataxia, and an absent β-lipoprotein.[10,153] Acanthocytes may be acquired in patients with severe hepatocellular disease (spur cells applied to that condition). A reduced serum cholesterol esterifying enzyme, lecithin:cholesterol acyltransferase (LCAT) is seen in patients with abetalipoproteinemia as well as in patients with liver disease who have either target cells or spur cells on smear.[165]

HEREDITARY SPHEROCYTOSIS

Key Words: Uniformly Sized Microspherocytes

Hereditary spherocytosis is an autosomal dominant trait characterized by the presence of uniformly sized microspherocytes on the peripheral blood smear, reticulocytosis (5–20%), an increased osmotic fragility of the rbcs in hypotonic saline, and a Type III hemolytic pattern in the autohemolysis test which is corrected by glucose.[187] The spleen plays an important role in the selective sequestration of these abnormal cells and splenectomy has a curative effect. The anemia is usually moderate with the MCV either normal or slightly reduced due to the presence of both microspherocytes and large polychromatophilic rbcs. The mean corpuscular hemoglobin concentration (MCHC) is either high normal or slightly increased because the hemoglobin is densely packed in microspherocytes which have lost more surface area than cellular contents by fragmentation. The defect in the rbcs in hereditary spherocytosis is intracorpuscular. There is an increased rigidity of the membrane of the rbcs with an increased permeability to the influx of sodium. The rbcs compensate for this leak by increasing the rate of transport of sodium out of the cell with a concomitant increase in glucose and ATP utilization. This mechanism is successful as long as there is sufficient glucose present.[94] However, in the spleen where erythrostasis occurs, glucose may fall to inadequate levels and ATP generation decreases and sodium leaks into the cell faster than it can be pumped out and swelling and lysis of the rbcs occurs.[96] There is also an excessive loss of membrane lipids which accounts for loss of surface area resulting in spherocyte formation since a spherocyte is formed when there is an alteration in the ratio of surface area to volume. Weed et al[178] have postulated that the rbc membrane may have an increased affinity for calcium resulting in a high intracellular calcium level which causes an actomyosin-like protein in the membrane to undergo a solid to gel transformation increasing cell rigidity. Jacob[94] feels that a microfilamentous membrane protein, spectrin, plays a role in the pathogenesis of the abnormal spherocyte. He has demonstrated that when normal rbcs are treated with vinblastine or heating erythrocytes are produced which mimic those in hereditary spherocytosis in all respects presumably through the denaturation of spectrin which is vital to rbc shape and deformity. Finally, the spleen in ideally suited to bring out the rbc defects in hereditary spherocytosis. When erythrostasis occurs, ATP depletion follows, leading to increased intracellular sodium, loss of membrane lipid, sphering, enhancement of calcium effect on membrane protein, alteration of spectrin, rigidity of membrane, and finally sequestration by the microcirculation of the spleen.[104]

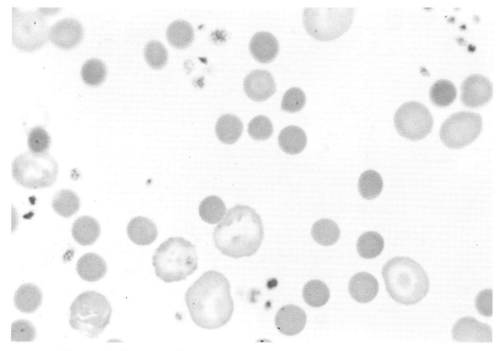

Figure 14.10.   Hereditary spherocytosis (original magnification ×600).

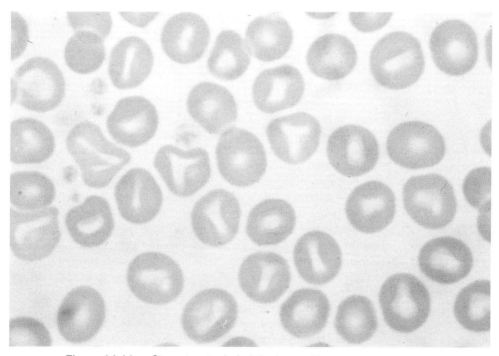

Figure 14.11.   Stomatocytosis (original magnification ×1050).

STOMATOCYTOSIS

Key Words: Slit-like Hypochromia, Defective Cation Pump

Stomatocytosis, erythrocytes with slit-like hypochromia, is associated with a chronic hemolytic process in which there is a marked increase in the passive leak of sodium into the erythrocyte and a marked increase in the potassium efflux due to defective cation pump.[76] Thus, stomatocytes have a high sodium level and a low potassium level as normally occurs in plasma. Normally the intracellular sodium level is low and the potassium level is high. Wiley et al in 1975[182] stressed the importance of rbc hydration in determining rbc morphology on dried smears. When the rbcs are overhydrated stomatocytes are plentiful, but when they are dehydrated, only target cells are seen on the dried smear, although bowl shapes appear in wet preparations. It is important to examine rbc morphology in both wet and dry states.

HEREDITARY ELLIPTOCYTOSIS

Hereditary elliptocytosis is an autosomal dominant trait.[39] In the majority of individuals this disorder follows a benign course, but 10–15% may show evidence of hemolysis or a frank hemolytic anemia.[132] The presence of spherocytes, schistocytes, burr cells, acanthocytes, and bizarre rbc shapes on the peripheral blood smear are morphologic indications of hemolysis. Small numbers of elliptical or oval rbcs may be seen in normal individuals and in a variety of hematologic dyscrasias, but not in the larger numbers that are seen in hereditary elliptocytosis.[9] Regularly greater than 25% of the rbcs are elliptical or oval and usually 50–90% may be seen.[9,186] The ovalocytes seen in B_{12}-folate deficiency may be distinguished from those seen in hereditary elliptocytosis by their macrocytic size.

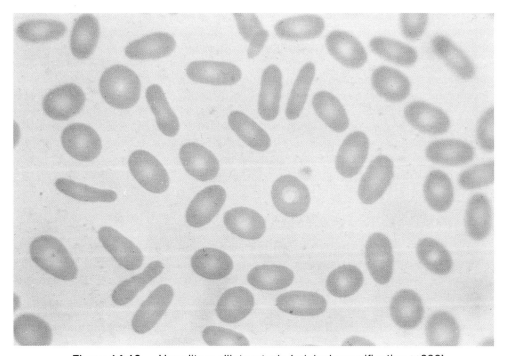

Figure 14.12.   Hereditary elliptocytosis (original magnification ×600).

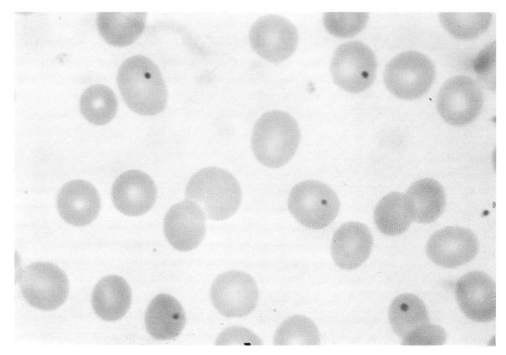

Figure 14.13. Postsplenectomy blood changes (original magnification ×1050).

POSTSPLENECTOMY BLOOD CHANGES

Howell-Jolly bodies are the most consistent finding in the blood in all patients following splenectomy and may persist for months and/or years.[186] Splenectomy results in changes in the morphology of the rbcs and in the concentration of platelets and leukocytes. The blood changes are similar after the removal of a normal spleen because of traumatic injury or the removal of the spleen for treatment of pathologic states. The most striking changes are seen in the rbcs. Nucleated rbcs, target cells, polychromatophilia (reticulocytosis), Pappenheimer bodies, and, of course, Howell-Jolly bodies are seen on the peripheral blood smear. Maximal leukocytosis occurs during the first postoperative week due to increased neutrophilia. Thrombocytosis occurs in approximately one-third of splenectomized patients and may also persist for months or years.[110]

ACUTE POSTHEMORRHAGIC ANEMIA

Anemia caused by an acute hemorrhage may be due to: 1) trauma; 2) ulcerative lesions of the gastrointestinal tract; 3) postoperative hemorrhage; 4) ruptured aneurysm; 5) ruptured ectopic pregnancy; 6) ruptured esophageal varices; or 7) spontaneous development or development after minor trauma in hemorrhagic disorders.[104]

The changes in the peripheral blood are dependent upon: 1) time elapsed since hemorrhage occurred; 2) the size and location of the hemorrhage; or 3) the nature of the underlying disease.[104]

The first changes probably noted on a peripheral blood smear following an acute hemorrhage is the presence of increased platelets and a neutrophilic leukocytosis.

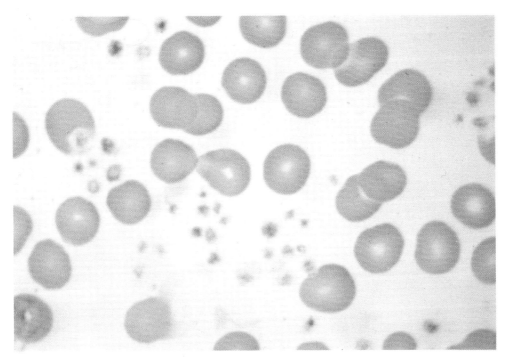

Figure 14.14.   Acute posthemorrhagic anemia (original magnification ×1050).

Platelet counts may approach 1,000,000/mm^3. The leukocyte count may reach 10,000–30,000/mm^3 within a few hours due to a shift of leukocytes from the marginal pools into the circulation and to the release of marrow granulocyte reserves.[186] Early neutrophilic forms, such as myelocytes, metamyelocytes, and some nucleated red blood cells, are only seen on the peripheral blood smear in severe hemorrhage accompanied by shock and tissue anoxia.

The degree of the anemia may not be apparent until 48–72 hours after the hemorrhage, the time for the hematocrit to reach its lowest point. The anemia is usually of the normocytic, normochromic type unless a preceding iron deficiency or strong reticulocytosis is present. Reticulocyte counts as high as 12–14% often follow an acute hemorrhage severe enough to reduce the red blood count to 3.0 million/mm.[3,67,104]

If bleeding has ceased, the erythrocyte count usually returns to normal in about 4 weeks, but the hemoglobin, with its vital oxygen-carrying capacity, does not return to normal levels until approximately 8 weeks posthemorrhage.[186]

SICKLE CELL ANEMIA

Sickle cell hemoglobin differs from normal hemoglobin in that the β-polypeptide chain contains valine in the sixth position where glutamic acid is found in normal hemoglobin, causing an electrophoretic difference in mobility of these hemoglobins.[91] The typical patient with sickle cell anemia is seen with a normochromic, normocytic anemia, if there are no overlying complications, in which the hemoglobin and red blood cell count are reduced to about one-half normal values.[104] The number and character of sickle cells on peripheral blood smears in patients with sickle cell anemia may not be sufficiently striking to warrant a diagnosis. However, in some cases of sickle cell crisis,

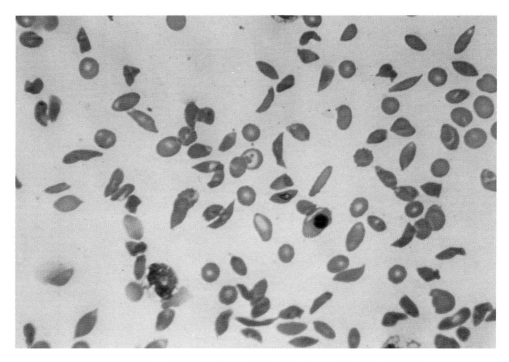

Figure 14.15.   Sickle cell anemia (original magnification ×600).

the crescent forms are plentiful.[184] Furthermore, sickled cells are rarely, if ever, seen in blood smears from persons with sickle cell trait.[72] The intracorpuscular defect in the globin portion of the hemoglobin molecule is responsible for the hemolytic nature of the anemia which is evidenced on smear by the finding of the poikilocytes of hemolysis: spherocytes, schistocytes, burr cells, and acanthocytes, and the signs of active red blood cell regeneration: Howell-Jolly bodies, nucleated rbcs, and polychromatophilia.[187] Reticulocytosis, in fact, exceeds 20%. Target cells are quite prominent on smears of sickle cell anemia patients as well. The leukocyte count is usually between 12,000–16,000/mm.[3] The platelet count is usually normal but counts over 1 million/mm^3 sometimes occur.[104]

The available screening tests for the detection of sickle cell hemoglobin are: the classic sickle cell preparation utilizing 2% sodium metabisulfite to induce deoxygenation of hemoglobin for sickling to occur; the solubility test which is dependent upon the decreased solubility of deoxygenated hemoglobin S in high phosphate buffer solution; and hemoglobin (Hb) electrophoresis. The most reliable methodology is probably electrophoresis utilizing cellulose acetate. The sickle cell preparation utilizing a reducing agent is not specific for Hb S since Hb C^{Harlem},[21] Hb C^{Georgetown},[138] Hb I,[3,154] and large amounts of Hb Barts[109] can also exhibit the sickling phenomenon.[183] The solubility test is hampered by the reliability of the commercially available kits which range from excellent to poor and because the cost of commercial products is prohibitive in laboratories doing high volume testing for sickle cell anemia.

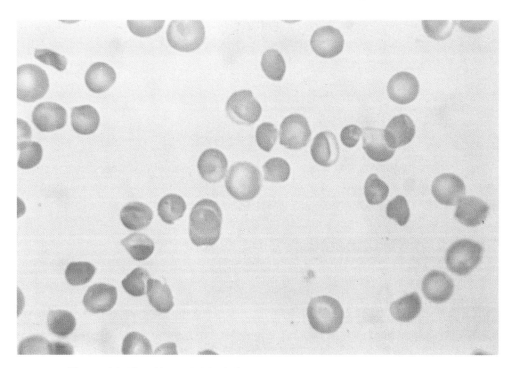

Figure 14.16.   Hemoglobin C-C disease (original magnification ×1050).

HEMOGLOBIN C DISEASE

In Hb C, lysine replaces glutamic acid in the sixth position of the β chain. Hb C occurs almost exclusively in blacks, in fact, Hb C trait is found in 2 or 3% of the Negro race.[169,187] The patients are characterized by splenomegaly and mild or moderately severe hemolytic anemia. The peripheral blood smear shows a normochromic, normocytic red blood cell population usually but occasionally the anemia is macrocytic in more severe cases. There are numerous target cells, microspherocytes, and slight to moderate numbers of envelope forms of which there are two types:

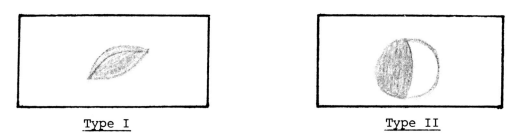

Type I   Type II

Type I which appears to be an erythrocyte folded over upon itself mimicking an envelope and also referred to as a "clam shell" or "clutch pocketbook" form. It is not seen exclusively in Hb C disease. It is also observed in Hb S disorders, thalassemia syndromes, and liver disease. Type II shows a concentration of hemoglobin to one side in the erythrocyte giving a flap-like appearance to the cell. Type II is also seen in the common hemoglobinopathies such as the sickling disorders and the thalassemia syndromes. Electron micrographs have shown tetragonal Hb C crystals in the hemoglobin portion of some of these cells. Although these envelope forms are not exclusive of Hb C and are seen in other conditions, their number is important. They are usually seen in moderate numbers in Hb C disease, persisting from field to field whereas in other conditions, their number is more occasional. A persistence of the Type II envelope form coupled to numerous target cells and easy to find microspherocytes in a normocytic, normochromic red blood cell population is strong morphologic evidence for the presence of Hb C disease.

Hb C may crystallize under conditions allowing partial drying or partial hemolysis and providing the concentration is greater than 44%.[33] Intraerythrocytic tetragonal crystals of Hb C have been observed in blood smears of patients with Hb C disorders.[47,181]

The Microcytic Anemias

IRON DEFICIENCY ANEMIA

The anemia of severe iron deficiency is characteristically hypochromic and microcytic. The mean corpuscular volume (MCV), mean corpuscular hemoglobin (MCH), and mean corpuscular hemoglobin concentration (MCHC) are all reduced in the typical patient. The average MCV is 74 fl (range, 53–93), MCHC 28 g/100 ml (range, 22–31), and MCH 20 pg (range, 14–29).[8,122] While the majority of red blood cells in patients with iron deficiency are smaller than normal with an increase in the central pallor (hypochromia), other erythrocytes appear normal in color and some show polychromatophilia if erythropoiesis is active.[104] The most common poikilocytes seen in iron deficiency are elongated or elliptical and tailed rbc forms.[187] Frequently burr cells are seen. Occasionally nucleated rbcs are observed. The leukocyte, platelet, and reticulocyte counts are usually normal.

In patients with mild or early iron deficiency, the anemia is not always hypochromic, microcytic, but may be hypochromic, normocytic or normochromic, normocytic. In these patients other laboratory tests are needed to establish the diagnosis of iron deficiency:[104]

1. Serum iron: usually reduced less than 40 g/100 ml in iron deficiency. (normal 50–150).[104]
2. Latent iron binding capacity: increased 2–3 times normal in iron deficiency (normal 200–300 µg/100 ml).
3. Prussian blue iron stain of bone marrow: marked depletion of storage iron.
4. Transferrin saturation: less than 10% in iron deficiency.[104]
5. Free erythro protoporphyrin: increased in iron deficiency within 1–2 weeks following acute decrease in saturation of serum iron to less than 15%.[104]

It should be emphasized to the student that the development of iron deficiency occurs gradually according to the following sequence of events: 1) depleted iron stores in the bone marrow; 2) increased serum iron-binding capacity; 3) decreased serum iron level; 4) appearance of normochromic or slightly hypochromic anemia; 5) development of hypochromic, microcytic anemia.[104]

The reverse sequence is true when the deficiency is treated with oral iron therapy.

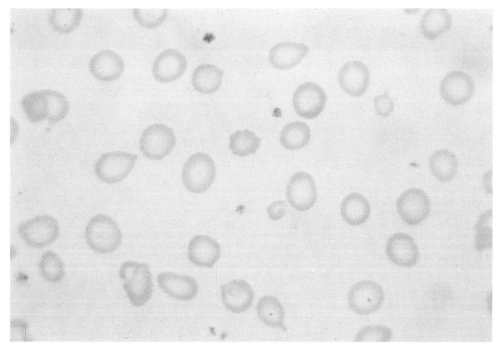

Figure 14.17.   Iron deficiency anemia (original magnification ×1050).

β THALASSEMIA MAJOR

Synonyms: Hereditary Leptocytosis, Cooley's Anemia, Mediterranean Anemia

Thalassemia major represents the homozygous inheritance of a biochemical defect in the synthesis of hemoglobin. There is no amino acid substitution and the hemoglobin, once formed, is normal in structure.[92] However, the synthesis of one of the polypeptide chains of hemoglobin is decreased or absent. The decrease in hemoglobin synthesis in thalassemia is thought to be due to a reduction in the messenger RNA that directs the synthesis of a specific hemoglobin chain.[15] A defect in the synthesis of the β chain is the most common type of thalassemia but defects in α, γ, and δ chains also occur.[176,177] There is a compensatory increase in hemoglobin F.

Thalassemia major is a microcytic hypochromic anemia which is usually severe. The peripheral blood smear shows marked poikilocytosis, anisocytosis, and polychromatophilia. The predominant poikilocyte is the leptocyte or target cell. The poikilocytes of hemolysis are also seen: acanthocytes, spherocytes, burr cells, and schistocytes. Moderate to marked basophilic strippling is seen in both the nucleated and non-nucleated forms of erythrocytes. Nucleated rbcs which are almost invariably present are often numerous and may outnumber the leukocytes. The last two nucleated rbc stages, the rubricyte and the metarubricyte, are the predominant forms seen. The first two nucleated stages of rbcs, the rubriblast and the prorubicyte, are rarely seen. Reticulocytosis is usually present and may be quite high, *e.g.*, 20% or greater. The signs of active normoblastic erythropoiesis are in evidence: Howell-Jolly bodies, polychromatophilia, and nucleated rbcs. Leukocyte counts range from 10,000–25,000/mm³, and occasionally an immature form is seen. Platelet counts are normal.[104,187]

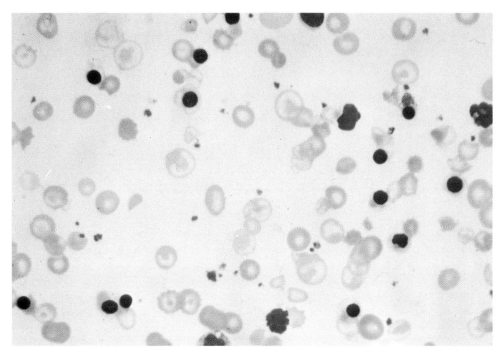

Figure 14.18.   Thalassemia major (original magnification ×600).

The finding of hypochromic microcytosis, target cells, late stage nucleated rbcs, basophilic stippling, poikilocytes of hemolysis: acanthocytes, spherocytes, burr cells, and schistocytes, and signs of active rbc regeneration: Howell-Jolly bodies, polychromatophilia, and nucleated rbcs is strong morphologic evidence for a diagnosis of thalassemia especially in a young person with hepatosplenomegaly and an increased hemoglobin F on electrophoresis.

β THALASSEMIA MINOR

Synonym: Thalassemia Trait

Thalassemia minor represents the heterozygous inheritance of a biochemical defect resulting in a decreased production of one of the polypeptide chains in hemoglobin synthesis probably due to a reduction in messenger RNA. There is a compensatory increase in hemoglobin A_2. Normally the hemoglobin A_2 component is present in amounts of 1–3%. In thalassemia trait, the A_2 level ranges from 3–7% with a mean of 5%.[102] In some cases of thalassemia minor, there is an increase in hemoglobin F rather than A_2 and this probably represents a variant.[177] However, unlike thalassemia major, the homozygous inheritance of this defect, the anemia in thalassemia minor is not severe. Most individuals are seen with a hemoglobin level only 1 or 2 g below normal and are in a reasonably good state of health. Individuals with thalassemia minor are discovered accidentally during examination in a doctor's office or in the hospital for unrelated causes, in a hemoglobin screening program, or in a family study. These patients are first suspected in a hematology laboratory when the Coulter S profile reveals a decreased MCV which is usually 64.70 ± 4.35 fl (range 52–75 fl). In our laboratory a hemoglobin electrophoresis is performed on all blood samples with MCVs

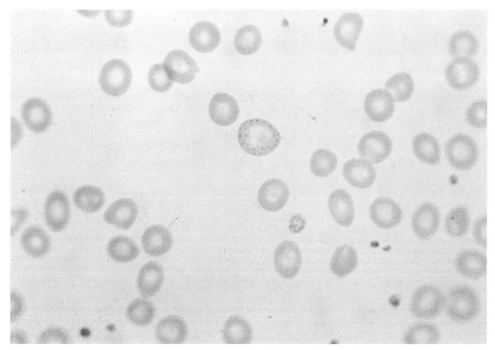

Figure 14.19.   Thalassemia minor (original magnification ×1050).

of 75 fl or less.[187] The anemia, when present, is microcytic, hypochromic and has often been confused with iron deficiency in the past. Thalassemia minor, however, is refractory to iron therapy. Because the typical erythrocytes are flat (leptocytes, target cells), they may appear normal in diameter and hypochromic even though the indices suggest that they are microcytic, normochromic. However, it has been my experience that in most cases of thalassemia minor the erythrocytes do appear to be microcytic whereas the hypochromia and the targeting of the rbcs is not as reliable since it is seen in fewer cases. Next to microcytosis, I weigh the finding of basophilic stippling of the rbcs most helpful. In some cases, the stippling is readily apparent whereas in other cases one must make a careful 5-minute scan to discover its presence. For cases of mild microcytic anemia, I usually instruct my students to make a 5-minute scan for basophilic stippling. The finding of five stippled rbcs in 5 minutes is strongly suggestive of thalassemia trait rather than mild iron deficiency since stippling is not usually seen in iron deficiency to that degree if at all. One must also consider sideroblastic anemia and lead poisoning in cases of microcytic hypochromia and basophilic stippling.

SIDEROBLASTIC ANEMIAS

The sideroblastic anemias are a heterogeneous group of acquired and inherited disorders which are characterized by excessive iron-overload in the mitochondria of normoblasts due to defective heme synthesis.[183] The perinuclear position of the iron-laden mitochondria is responsible for the "ringed" sideroblast seen on Prussian blue-stained smears of the bone marrow. The term "sideroblast," therefore, refers to a nucleated red blood cell with deposition of iron granules and a "siderocyte" refers to a non-nucleated red blood cell containing iron granules. "Pappenheimer bodies" is the term used to imply iron granules in red blood cells on Wright's-stained smears based on

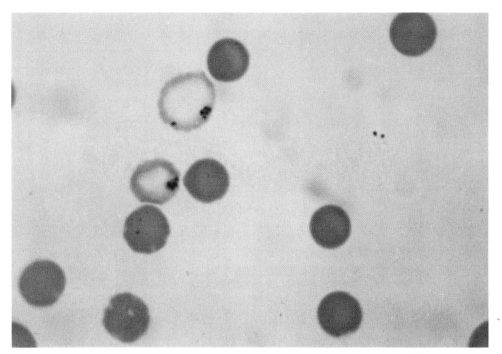

Figure 14.20. Sideroblastic anemia (original magnification ×1500).

their morphologic appearance. Pappenheimer bodies are usually found in one or two small closely aggregated clusters in erythrocytes which distinguishes them from the evenly dispersed arrangement of precipitated RNA or basophilic stippling also found in these cells.

In the classic hereditary form of sideroblastic anemia, there is a moderately severe hypochromic, microcytic anemia (MCV 53–68 fl, MCH 18–20 pg, and MCHC 33%).[104] However, in some cases, hereditary sideroblastic anemia is normocytic or macrocytic. Normocytic or macrocytic anemia is more frequently found in the acquired form of sideroblastic anemia (MCV 80–114 fl). A striking morphologic feature of the erythrocytes in sideroblastic anemia patients is dimorphism in which some of the erythrocytes possess the normal amount of hemoglobin while others are hypochromic.[187] The hypochromic cells will vary greatly in size and shape. The hemoglobin level is usually between 7–10 g/100 ml, but it may be as low as 3 g/100 ml.[183] Increased numbers of siderocytes, schistocytes, target cells, spherocytes, and even nucleated red blood cells may be seen. Reticulocyte counts are usually normal or slightly increased. Occasionally a reticulocyte count as high as 15% is encountered.[104]

The leukocyte count is normal or low and when decreased may be accompanied by neutropenia. Occasionally an early myeloid form (*e.g.*, myelocyte) is seen on the peripheral blood smear. Normal monocytes may be increased.

Platelets are usually normal but thrombocytosis and thrombocytopenia have both occurred in some patients.

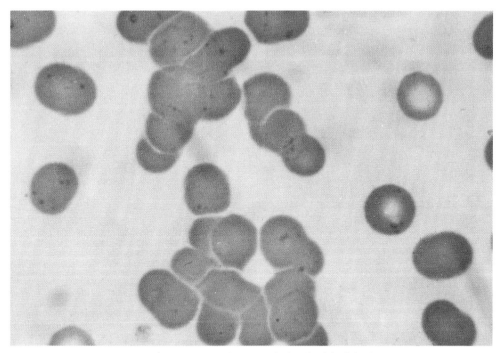

Figure 14.21.   Cold agglutinin disease (true agglutination) (original magnification ×1500).

Cold Agglutinin Disease and Rouleaux Formation

COLD AGGLUTININ DISEASE (TRUE AGGLUTINATION)

Cold autoantibodies to rbc antigens react best under 32°C and are responsible for two clinical syndromes: 1) cold agglutinin syndrome, the most common, responsible for one-third of all cases of autoimmune hemolytic anemia and seen in association with infections (*Mycoplasma pneumoniae*[95]), malignancy, or occasionally in the absence of underlying disease, 2) the rare paroxysmal cold hemoglobinuria due to hemolysins found in congenital or acquired syphilis.[187] Cold agglutinins form rbc clumps which are more irregularly distributed throughout the microscopic field than rouleaux formation and vary more in size. The rbcs adhere to each other at all angles giving a "grape-like" clusters in cold agglutinin syndrome which is not disrupted by the addition of saline unless the titer is at a critically low level whereas rouleaux formation is dispersed upon addition of saline.[156]

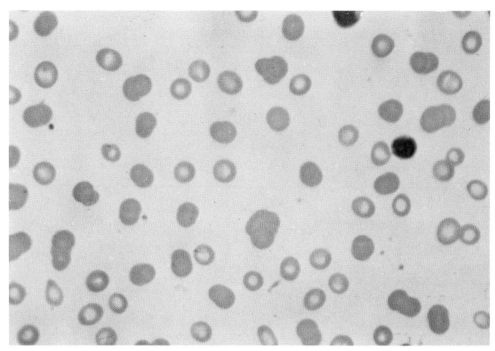

Figure 14.22.   Rouleaux formation (pseudoagglutination) (original magnification ×600).

ROULEAUX FORMATION (PSEUDOAGGLUTINATION)[40]

Marked rouleaux formation of the rbcs may be seen in patients whose serum contains high concentrations of abnormal globulins or fibrinogen, *e.g.*, multiple myeloma, Waldenstrom's macroglobulinemia, or cryoglobulinemia, etc.). Small rouleaux formations are characteristically fairly evenly spaced throughout the microscopic field and do not vary greatly in size. In rouleaux formation, the rbcs exhibit side to side adherence giving a short "stacked coin" appearance with the flat surfaces being exposed.[183] The dilution of serum with saline inhibits rouleaux formation whereas true agglutination is not affected unless the titer is at a critically low level.

Chapter 15

Erythrocyte Inclusion Bodies

Howell-Jolly Bodies

1. These are small spherical basophilic bodies usually no larger than 1 μm in diameter seen in erythrocytes.[121] They usually occur singly but occasionally occur in multiple.[183]
2. In pathologic conditions, they are thought to represent a chromosome separated from the mitotic spindle during abnormal mitosis.[100] Under normal conditions, they are believed to be derived from nuclear fragmentation (karyorrhexis) or incomplete nuclear expulsion. In either case, they represent a small nuclear remnant which gives a positive Feulgen reaction for DNA and are most commonly seen following splenectomy, in hemolytic anemia, in megaloblastic anemia, and in hyposplenism.[49,183]

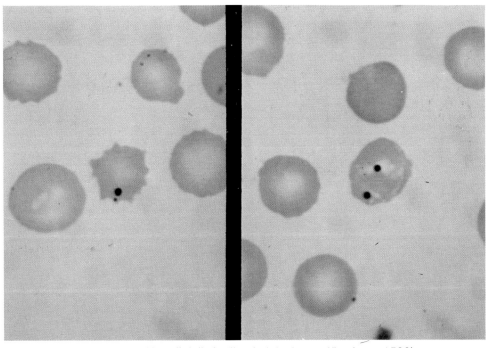

Figure 15.1   Howell–Jolly bodies (original magnification ×1500).

Pappenheimer Bodies (Wright's Stain) or Siderotic Granules (Prussian Blue Stain)

1. These are small irregular basophilic inclusions seen in erythrocytes.[70,71] They are called Pappenheimer bodies when viewed on Wright's-stained smears[121] and siderotic granules or siderosomes when they are seen on Prussian blue-stained smears which confirms that they are iron particles.[134]

2. Nucleated red blood cells containing Pappenheimer bodies are called sideroblasts and non-nucleated red blood cells with Pappenheimer bodies are called siderocytes.[40]

3. These inclusions must be differentiated from punctate basophilia or "stippling" and can usually be distinguished by their irregular size and shape but mostly by their tendency to aggregate in small clusters within the erythrocyte usually near the periphery of the cell. Basophilic stippling tends to be uniform in size and shape and is usually evenly dispersed throughout the erythrocyte.[40]

4. Pappenheimer bodies are seen in severe hemolytic anemia, splenic atrophy, post-splenectomy, sideroblastic anemia, thalassemia, chloramphenicol toxicity, and occasionally in B_{12} or folate deficiency.[31,126,183]

5. In normal subjects, 30–50% of the red blood cell precursors are sideroblasts. The inclusions are small, few in number (usually less than five),[54] and are not ringed around the nucleus. Pathologic sideroblasts contain larger, more numerous (greater than five), and commonly are found "ringed" around the nucleus. These "ringed" sideroblasts are found only in pathologic circumstances, usually in the sideroblastic anemias. Electron microscopy shows these inclusions to be mitochondria containing ferruginous micelles in pathologic states rather than ferritin aggregates which characterize normal siderocytes.[17,18,24]

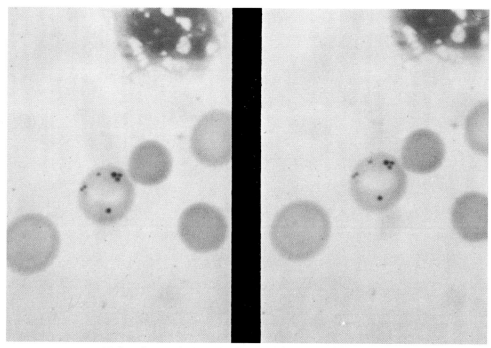

Figure 15.2.   Pappenheimer bodies (original magnification ×1500).

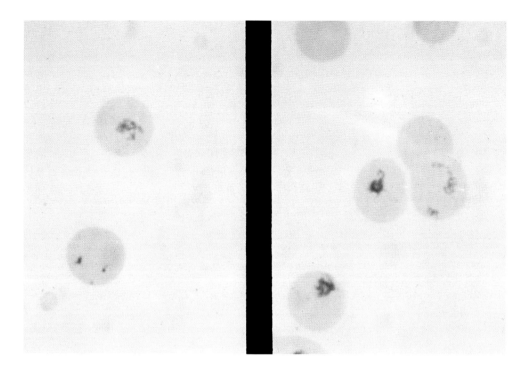

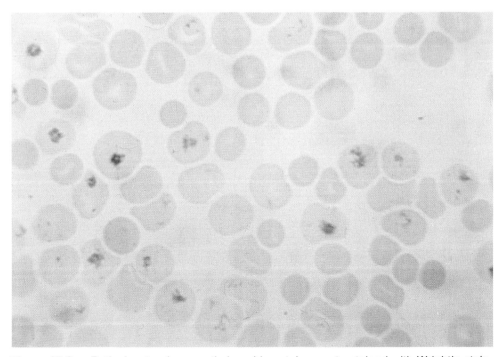

Figure 15.3.   Reticulocytes (new methylene blue stain counterstained with Wright's stain. *Upper*, original magnification ×1500. *Lower*, original magnification ×600. (For description, see next page.)

Reticulocytes

1. Reticulocytes are immature red blood cells which contain remnants of the basophilic ribonucleoprotein (RNA) which was present in larger amounts in the cytoplasm of the nucleated precursors of this cell line.[40] The least mature reticulocytes are those with the largest amount of precipitate and the most mature reticulocytes contain only a few dots or short strands of same. The formation of basophilic ribonucleoprotein (RNA) into a reticulum takes place only in vitally or supravitally stained unfixed preparations. New methylene blue N Color Index No. 52030 is superior to brilliant cresyl blue Color Index No. 51010 because of its uniform performance and intense blue staining of the reticulum.[31]

2. Reticulocytes are slightly larger than mature erythrocytes measuring 9–10 μm in diameter as compared to the 6–8 μm size of normal red blood cells.[183,187]

3. The number of reticulocytes in the peripheral blood is an index of erythropoietic activity with higher values being indicative of bleeding or hemolysis. Reticulocytes are usually expressed as the number per 100 red blood cells. Normally 0.5–2% reticulocytes are seen.[183,186]

4. Siderotic granules and basophilic stippling also stain blue with new methylene blue N and brilliant cresyl blue and cannot be distinguished from reticulocytes so are therefore included in reticulocyte counts. Heinz bodies and Howell-Jolly bodies also stain blue with these dyes but can usually be distinguished by their morphology.[31]

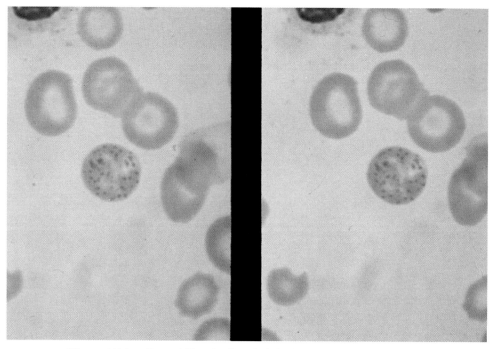

Figure 15.4.   Basophilic stippling (original magnification ×1500).

Basophilic Stippling

1. "Punctate basophilia" or "stippling" is fine or coarse evenly dispersed bluish or bluish black granules found in erythrocytes.
2. Basophilic stippling is a reflection of immaturity and the persistence of ribose nucleoprotein (RNA) in the erythrocyte. Electron microscopy confirms the inclusions as agglutinated or clumped ribosomes.[97,98,173]
3. Diffuse or fine stippling is seen in a variety of anemias. Coarse stippling is seen after exposure to lead and other metals, in thalassemia, and is associated with defective heme synthesis.[183]

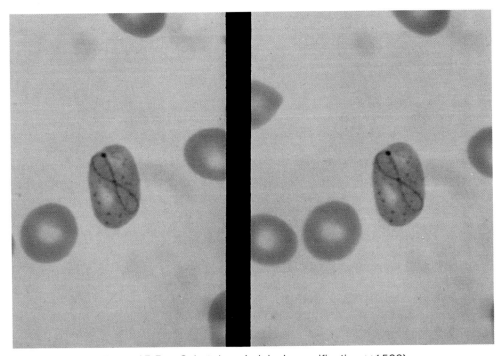

Figure 15.5.   Cabot rings (original magnification ×1500).

Cabot Rings

1. Single or double rings, stippled "necklace"-shaped loops, and "figure eight" loops which can occur in both nucleated and non-nucleated erythrocytes. They are commonly seen in association with coarse stippling in these cells.[99]
2. They may appear basophilic or acidophilic on Wright's-stained smears in patients with severe anemia especially untreated pernicious anemia, following splenectomy, and leukemia. Many investigators consider these inclusions an artifact.[99]
3. It is not certain whether Cabot rings represent remnants of nuclear material or products of cellular degeneration due to toxic substances. Cytochemical tests have shown the rings contain arginine-rich histone and non-hemoglobin iron and do not contain DNA.[49,78]

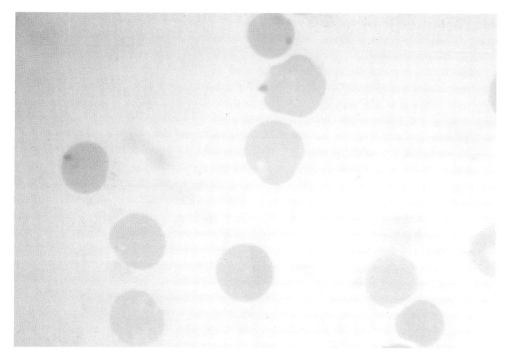

Figure 15.6.   Heinz bodies (original magnification ×1500); brilliant cresyl blue stain.

Heinz Bodies

1. Heinz bodies are deep blue-purple irregularly shaped inclusions which measure 0.3–2 μm in diameter by light microscopy. One or more may be seen in an erythrocyte. They are usually eccentrically placed and often attach to the rbc membrane. They may protrude from the erythrocyte or occur free in plasma.

2. Heinz bodies represent precipitated, denatured hemoglobin due to oxidative injury by oxidant drugs, *e.g.*, nitro and/or amine compounds and also occur in individuals with hereditary defects in the hexose-monophosphate shunt, such as glucose 6-phosphodiesterase deficiency, α thalassemia, unstable hemoglobins and in splenectomized patients.

3. Heinz bodies may be seen in fresh wet unstained preparations of blood where they appear as globular refractile bodies.[31] Heinz bodies are not visible in Wright's-stained preparations of blood since both normal and denatured hemoglobin stain pink with this Romanowsky dye and are indistinguishable. They do stain with crystal violet or methyl violet and with brilliant cresyl blue and new methylene blue.

4. Electron microscopic studies depict inability of rigid Heinz bodies to traverse interepithelial slits of the splenic sinus and, therefore, these inclusion bodies are left behind in the perisinusoidal red pulp for phagocytosis by macrophages of the reticuloendothelial system.[107] Electron microscopic studies also reveal that Heinz bodies originate as dense masses in the center of the red blood cell and then attach to the membrane of the cell.[148,149,184]

Chapter 16

Problems in Interpreting Red Blood Cell Morphology

Dacryocytes (Teardrop Red Blood Cell and Tailed Red Blood Cell)

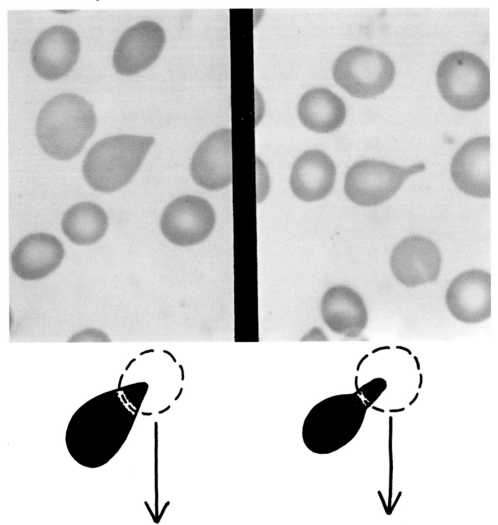

Figure 16.1. *Upper,* teardrop red blood cell (*left*), *versus* tailed red blood cell (*right*). *Lower,* schematic diagram. Teardrop rbc (*left*), rbc with shorter projection than that of the tailed rbc which exhibits a lessening of the cellular diameter terminating in point. Tailed rbc (*right*), rbc with elongated projection with rounded end and constant diameter maintained from beginning to end.

207

Sickle Cell and Envelope Form

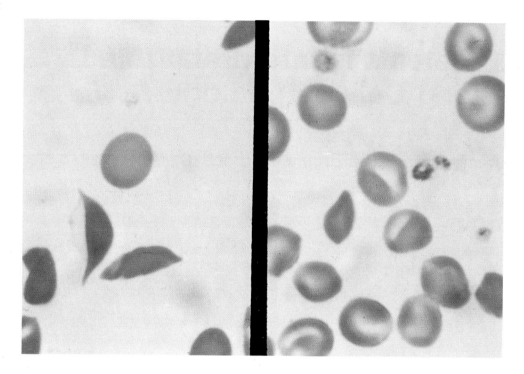

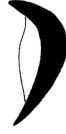

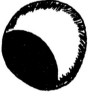

Figure 16.2.   *Upper*, Sickle cell (drepanocyte) (*left*) *versus* the envelope form (*right*). *Lower*, schematic diagram. Sickle cell (drepanocyte) (*left*). 1) This rbc form represents the molecular aggregation of S hemoglobin. 2) This is the filamentous form of sickle cell. The envelope form (*right*). 1) This rbc form may represent the precipitation of tetragonal crystals of C hemoglobin; 2) Moderate numbers of these forms are seen in hemoglobin C disease but slight numbers are seen in thalassemia major, liver disease, and sickle cell anemia.

Spherocyte and Acanthocyte

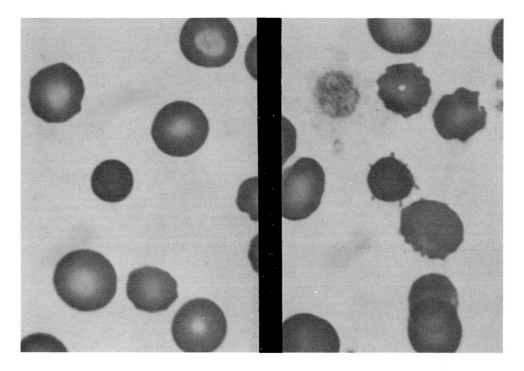

Figure 16.3. *Upper,* Spherocyte (*left*) *versus* acanthocyte (*right*). *Lower,* schematic diagram. Spherocyte (*left*). 1) Intensely stained rbc (bright red-orange) with no central pallor containing a high hemoglobin concentration with a low to normal cellular volume (surface/volume ratio is decreased). 2) *No* oblique projections noted. Acanthocyte (*right*). 1) Intensely stained rbc (bright red-orange) with no central pallor containing a high hemoglobin concentration with a low to normal cellular volume (surface/volume ratio is decreased). 2) Spherocyte with 2–10 oblique projections[184] noted.

Sickle Cells (Drepanocytes)

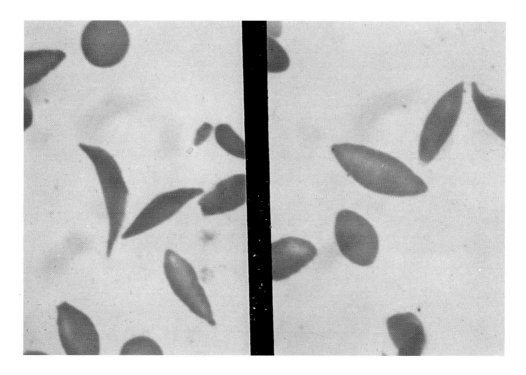

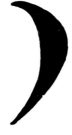

Figure 16.4. *Upper,* the filamentous form (*left*) *versus* the oat cell form (*right*). *Lower,* schematic diagram. Filamentous form (*left*): 1) irreversible upon oxygenation; 2) half-moon or crescent shape to cell with center cell diameter narrow; 3) more distinct points at each end of cell. Oat cell form (*right*): 1) reversible upon oxygenation; 2) straight appearance to cell with center cell diameter broader than filamentous form; 3) Less distinct points at each end of cell.

Acanthocyte *versus* Keratocyte (Burr Cell)

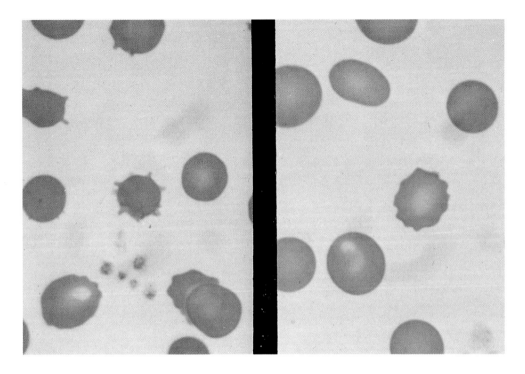

Figure 16.5.   *Upper,* acanthocyte *(left) versus* the keratocyte (burr cell) *(right). Lower,* schematic diagram. Acanthocyte *(left):* 1) must be a spherocyte; 2) exhibits 2–10 sharp oblique, irregularly spaced projections which vary in width and length[184]; 3) refer to acanthocyte *versus* spherocyte on page 209. Keratocyte (burr cell) *(right):* 1) is usually a normocyte; 2) blunt, evenly spaced projections (10–30) at the cellular periphery; 3) slight central pallor usually noted.

Sickle Cell *versus* Schistocyte (Schizocyte)

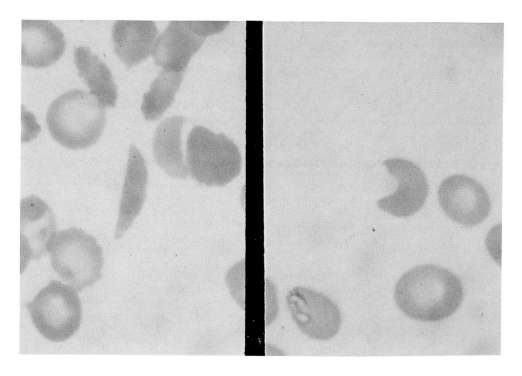

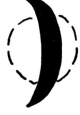

Figure 16.6.   *Upper*, sickle cell (drepanocyte) (left) *versus* schistocyte (schizocyte) (*right*). *Lower*, schematic diagram. Sickle cell (Drepanocyte) (*left*). 1) The filamentous form of the sickle cell elongates beyond the circumference of a normal sized rbc. 2) Center diameter of cell is usually more narrow than that of the schistocyte. Schistocyte (Schizocyte) (*right*). 1) The helmet cell form of schistocyte pictured above does *not* usually elongate beyond the circumference of a normal sized rbc. 2) The center diameter of the cell is broader than the filamentous form of sickle cell.

Elliptocyte *versus* Sickle Cell (Filamentous Form)

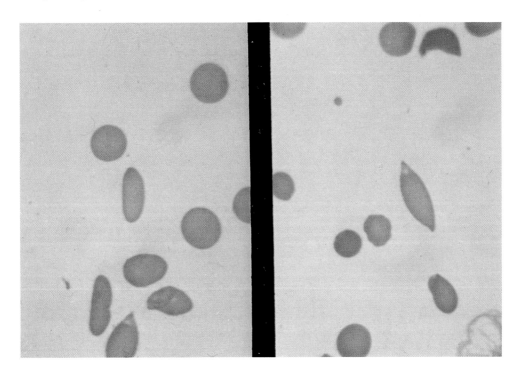

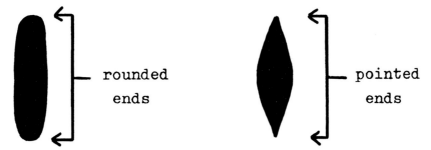

Figure 16.7. *Upper,* Elliptocyte (*left*) *versus* sickle cell (drepanocyte) (filamentous form) (*right*). *Lower,* schematic diagram. Elliptocyte (*left*): 1) elongated red blood cell with *rounded ends;* 2) cellular diameter appears equivocal from top to bottom. Sickle cell (drepanocyte) (filamentous form) (*right*): 1) elongated red blood cell with *pointed ends;* 2) cellular diameter is broad in center of cell and narrows toward the ends of the cell into a point.

Blister Cell *versus* Helmet Cell Form (Schistocyte)

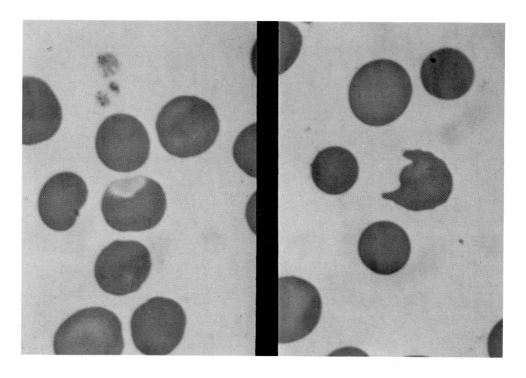

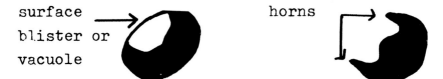

Figure 16.8. *Upper,* blister cell form (*left*) *versus* helmet cell form (schistocyte) (interme-diate form) (*right*). *Lower,* schematic diagram. A surface blister or vacuole devoid of hemoglobin forms near the cell periphery (*left*). The vacuole enlarges causing the red cell membrane to rupture leaving two horns which give the cell a half-moon shape with a central crater effect. This is the intermediate cell or helmet cell (*right*) (a form of schistocyte). A flattening of the crater with further distortion produces the third form—the burr cell.

Chapter 17

Leukocyte Nuclear Appendages and Leukocyte Inclusion Bodies

Polymorphonuclear Leukocyte "Drumsticks" in Women

1. The "drumstick" appendage consists of an oval mass of dense chromatin 1.2–1.5 μm in size attached to a nuclear lobe by a single fine filament in neutrophils (most commonly), eosinophils, and probably basophils. It is representative of the sex chromatin body of these leukocytes in normal female blood but not normal male blood. It is seen in men with the XXY chromosome abnormality known as Klinefelter's syndrome and is absent in chromatin-negative women with Turner's syndrome.[45,114]

2. The incidence of drumsticks in normal female blood has been determined as 0.6–8.8% with a mean of 3.1%.[142]

3. The "drumstick" appendage must be distinguished from nonspecific nodules, such as small clubs, sessile nodules, minor lobes, tags, and racket formation.

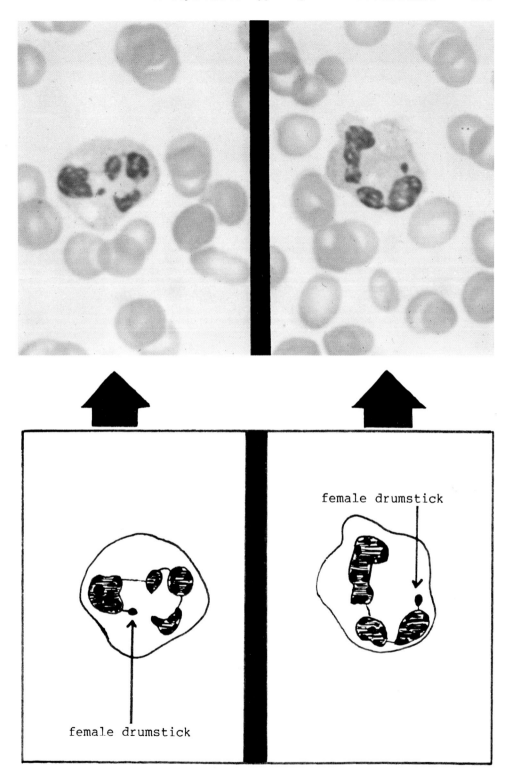

Figure 17.1. *Upper*, polymorphonuclear leukocyte "drumsticks" in females. *Lower*, schematic diagram.

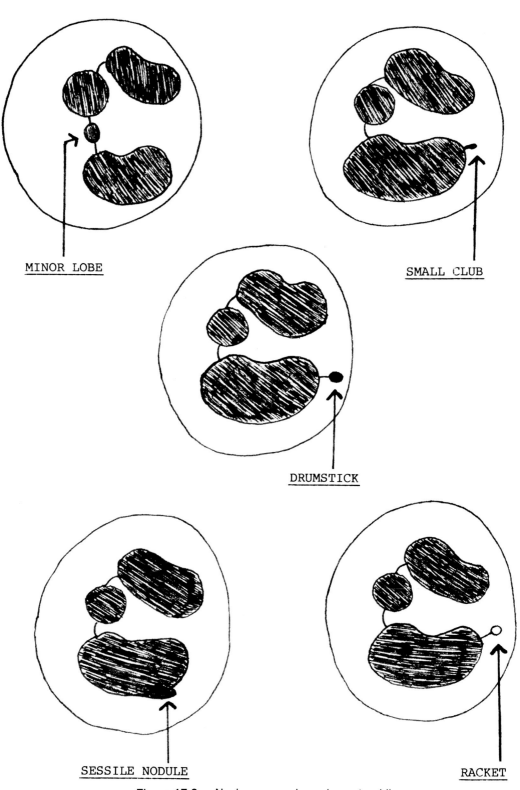

MINOR LOBE

SMALL CLUB

DRUMSTICK

SESSILE NODULE

RACKET

Figure 17.2.   Nuclear appendages in neutrophils.

Toxic Granulation

1. Toxic granulation is manifested by dark, basophilic granules found in the cytoplasm of late stage myeloid cells and monocytes which vary from fine to coarse in consistency and from few to numerous in number.
2. Electron microscopy and histochemical studies reveal that toxic granules are azurophilic (primary), peroxidase-positive inclusions.[120]
3. They are seen in severe infections, burns, or malignancy, or may be drug-induced.[66]

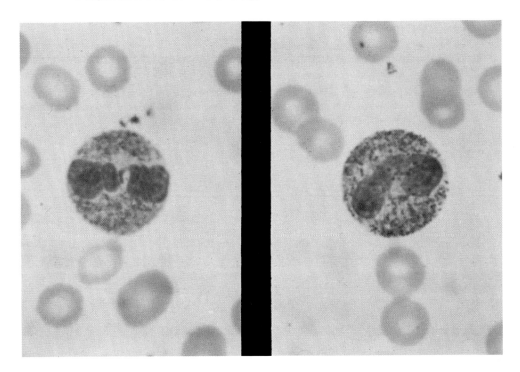

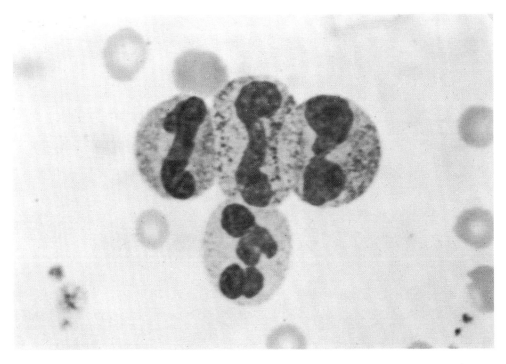

Figure 17.3.   Toxic granulation. *Upper*, segmented neutrophil and band neutrophil. *Lower*, original magnification ×1500.

Döhle Bodies

1. Döhle bodies are single or multiple round, oval, or filamentous sky-blue inclusions with Romanowksy stains found at the periphery of the cytoplasm of neutrophils. Döhle inclusions may also be seen in earlier myeloid cells, lymphocytes, and monocytes.[50,183]
2. Döhle bodies represent lamellar aggregates of rough endoplasmic reticulum according to electron microscopic studies.
3. They are associated with toxicity and may be seen together with toxic granulation in scarlet fever, severe infections, burns,[179] after administration of cytotoxic agents, *e.g.*, cyclophosphamide,[93] and uncomplicated pregnancy.
4. Döhle bodies must be differentiated from May-Hegglin bodies which are morphologically identical. Signs of toxicity, such as a shift to the left in the myeloid series, elevated total leukocyte count, or toxic granulation and/or vacuolization in the cytoplasm of myeloid cells, suggest Döhle bodies whereas a normal total leukocyte count, no shift to the left, the presence of giant abnormal platelets, or lack of toxic granulation of neutrophils suggests May-Hegglin anomaly.
5. Döhle-like inclusions may be seen in the rare Chediak-Higashi syndrome.

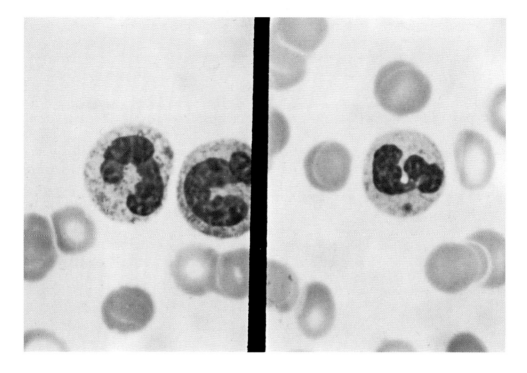

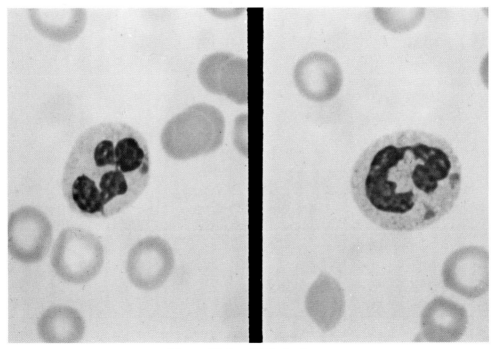

Figure 17.4.   Döhle bodies.

Auer Rods

1. Auer rods are pink-staining rod-shaped inclusions measuring 0.1–2 μm in breadth and 3–6 μm in length which are found in the cytoplasm of immature cells of myeloblastic, myelomonocytic, or monocytic leukemia.[31] The presence of Auer rods excludes lymphocytic leukemia.[31,142]
2. Auer rods appear to be lysosomal in nature and represent a fusion of cytoplasmic granules into a crystalline plaque or rod.[62]
3. These inclusions are peroxidase-positive and contain acid phosphatase and esterase.[60,65,74]

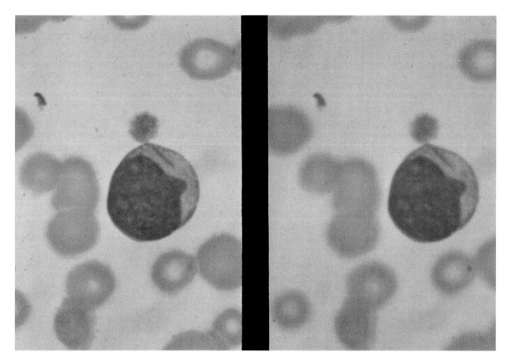

Figure 17.5.   Auer rods in blast cell.

Chapter 18

Leukocytes in Disease

Acute Granulocytic Leukemia

The peripheral blood film in a patient with acute granulocytic leukemia is usually characterized by a predominance of blast cells. It is difficult to differentiate leukoblasts (myeloblasts, lymphoblasts, monoblasts) by current methodology: morphology, histochemical staining, electron microscopy. However, the greatest contribution to the identification of blast cells is made by noting the cellular company they keep; in other words, the more mature and easily recognized cells on the same smear, *e.g.,* promyelocytes, myelocytes, metamyelocytes. When the blast cells are associated with promyelocytes containing obvious azurophilic primary granulation with Wright's stain, this is strong presumptive evidence that the blast forms are granulocytic in origin. The presence of Auer rods (acidophilic, rod-shaped inclusions) in the cytoplasm of the immature cells is pathognomonic of granulocytic or monocytic leukemia. Unfortunately, they are found in only 5–10% of cases.[183] The number of nucleoli in the nucleus of blast forms is helpful since lymphoblasts usually show 1–2 nucleoli whereas myeloblasts can show 1–5 nucleoli per nucleus.[187]

The leukocyte count is elevated in approximately 50% of the patients.[187] In patients with normal or decreased leukocyte counts, blast cells are still in evidence on the peripheral blood smear. Less than 20% of patients have with leukocyte counts of 100,000/mm^3 or greater and rarely a leukocyte count of 1,000,000/mm^3 may be observed.[186]

A moderate to severe normochromic, normocytic anemia is usually seen in these patients. Occasional nucleated red blood cells may be observed in the peripheral blood. Increased numbers of nucleated red blood cells in all stages of development (20 or more per 100 leukocytes) would be strongly suggestive of Di Guglielmo's syndrome, a variant of acute granulocytic leukemia.[161] Reticulocytes are usually decreased. This is a reflection of decreased cellular production.

A moderate to severe thrombocytopenia is an important additional finding in patients with acute granulocytic leukemia and is usually present at the time of diagnosis. Rarely, thrombocytosis is seen.[4]

Occasionally a case of acute granulocytic leukemia is seen in which there is a high prevalence of blast forms which keep company with increased numbers of band neutrophils and segmented neutrophils and the intermediate forms (promyelocytes, myelocytes, metamyelocytes) are conspicuous by their absence. This gap or hiatus of the intermediate forms has led to the term "hiatus leukemicus" for this unusual form of acute granulocytic leukemia. If one conducts a careful scan of the peripheral blood film for several minutes, an isolated myelocyte or metamyelocyte can usually be found.

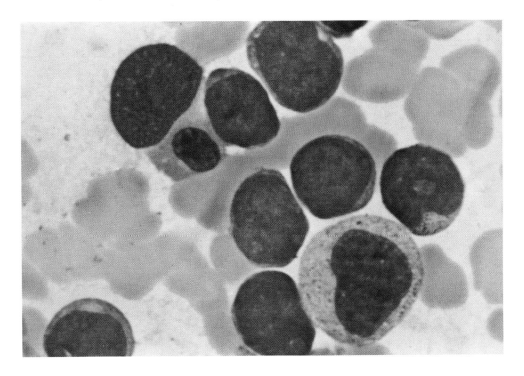

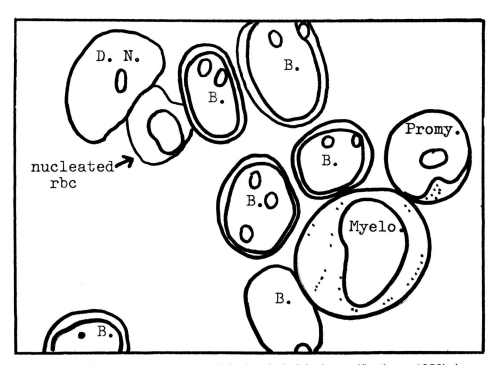

Figure 18.1. *Upper*, acute granulocytic leukemia (original magnification ×1050). *Lower*, schematic diagram. D. N., degenerative nucleus; B., blast cell; Promy., promyelocyte; Myelo., myelocyte.

Acute Promyelocytic Leukemia

The diagnosis of acute promyelocytic leukemia (APL) may be determined by the presence of promyelocytes containing abnormally prominent primary granules.[20] The relative number of promyelocytes is of little importance, in fact, Rosenthal[151] reported that myeloblasts were generally greater in number than promyelocytes in his cases of APL. However, blast and promyelocyte forms are the predominant myeloid stages seen in APL with the more mature myeloid forms conspicuously reduced or absent whereas in subacute myelogenous leukemia, in which the promyelocyte may be predominant, the more mature myeloid stages are readily apparent and the promyelocytes are normal morphologically.

The prominent leukemic cell in APL is an atypical or abnormal promyelocyte in which the nucleus may appear more immature than in the normal promyelocyte with very fine chromatin and prominent nucleoli. The granules may be normal in appearance but frequently are quite large and oval rather than round and have variable staining characteristics. The cytoplasm may be abundant and is relatively mature with little basophilia in some cases of APL. Branched or adherent Auer rods are common.[187]

Eighty to 90% of the cases of APL have hemorrhagic manifestations characterized by hypofibrinogenemia and disseminated intravascular coagulation (DIC).[11, 151] The clotting probably results from the release of material with tissue thromboplastin activity from the granules of the leukemic cells.[183] DIC abnormalities are correlated with the presence of the large abnormal granules rather than myeloblast to promyelocyte ratio.

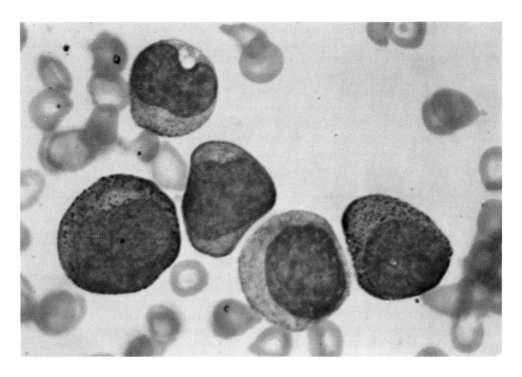

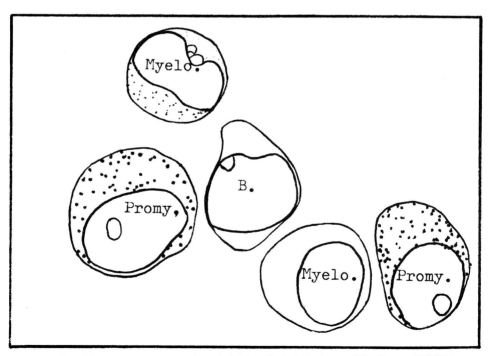

Figure 18.2.   *Upper*, acute promyelocytic leukemia (original magnification ×1500). *Lower*, schematic diagram. *B*; blast cell; *Promy*; promyelocyte; *Myelo.*, myelocyte.

Chronic Granulocytic Leukemia

The diagnosis of chronic granulocytic leukemia can usually be made at a glance when one examines the peripheral blood smear of most patients due to the striking granulocytic leukocytosis and the marked outpouring of all stages of maturation. The leukocyte count is greater than 100,000/mm³ in 62[117]–90%[188] of patients at the time of diagnosis and may exceed 1,000,000/mm³ in some cases.[117] In most instances, however, the leukocyte count is between 100,000–300,000/mm³. Myelocytes and later stages of development (metamyelocytes, band cells, segmented neutrophils) predominate in the peripheral blood smear of these patients. A few myeloblasts and promyelocytes may be seen, but they constitute a small percentage of the cells (usually less than 10%) until a blastic crisis ensues which is usually the terminal event in this disorder. The absolute number of basophils is increased as are eosinophils with early stages of these acidophilic cells in evidence frequently.[186]

A mild normochromic, normocytic anemia is present at diagnosis in most patients with chronic granulocytic leukemia.[106] The number of reticulocytes is normal or slightly increased. Rarely, a hemolytic anemia is present.[116] Nucleated rbcs are occasionally seen in scanning blood films in chronic granulocytic leukemia, but they are rarely as numerous as they are in myeloid metaplasia.

The platelet count is increased in approximately 50% of patients.[117,188] Thrombocytosis may be excessive and it is not uncommon for counts to exceed 1,000,000/mm³ or even two to three times this level.[187] Severe thrombocytopenia is rare in typical cases at diagnosis but is seen later in the disease.

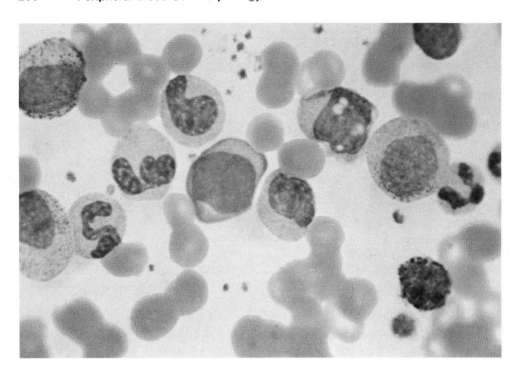

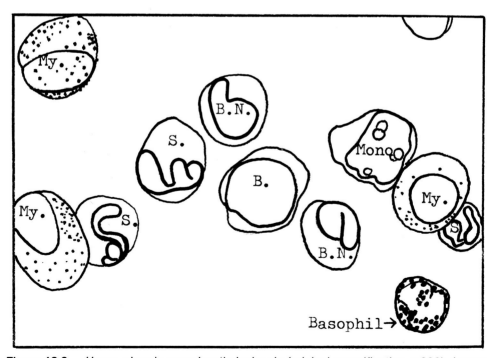

Figure 18.3. *Upper*, chronic granulocytic leukemia (original magnification ×600). *Lower*, schematic diagram. *My*., myelocyte; *B.N.*, band neutrophil; *S*., segmented neutrophil; *Mono*, monocyte; *B*., blast cell.

Basophilic Leukemia

The characteristic finding in basophilic leukemia is a predominance of basophilic leukocytes[103] on the peripheral blood smear of a patient with the clinical picture of leukemia which may be acute or chronic.[186] In the acute form, blast cells and promyelocytes are found with the basophilic leukocytes on the blood film. In acute cases, if there is a question as to whether the leukemic cells contain neutrophilic or basophilic granules, one can perform two histochemical stains to make the distinction: the toluidine blue stain and the peroxidase stain.[82] Basophilic granules would be positive with the toluidine blue stain and neutrophilic granules would be negative. Conversely, neutrophilic granules are peroxidase-positive and basophilic granules are peroxidase-negative. In the 40 cases of basophilic leukemia studied by Quatrin,[141] 20–40% basophilic leukocytes were found most frequently. Ten of these patients followed an acute course and succumbed in 4–6 weeks. They exhibited serious hemorrhagic manifestations which were probably associated with the increase in basophils with their heparin-containing granules. The cases of basophilic leukemia which have been classified as chronic have shown the picture of chronic myelogenous leukemia but with an extreme elevation in the basophil count. The classification of leukemia as basophilic is arbitrary, however, since a basophilic leukocytosis can be characteristic of chronic myelogenous leukemia. To distinguish some cases from basophilic leukemoid reactions, especially to tuberculosis, is also difficult.[87]

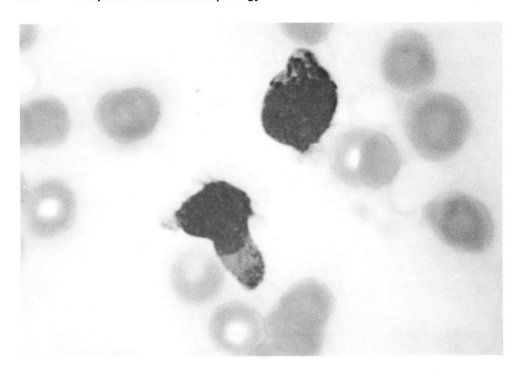

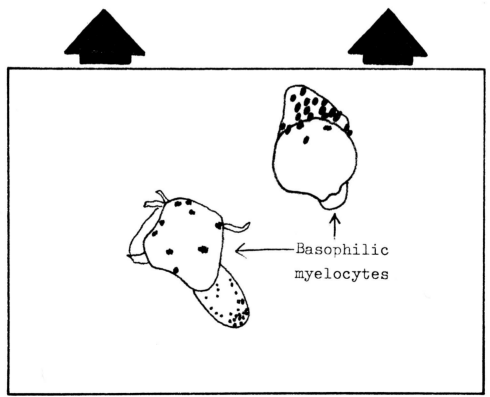

Figure 18.4. *Upper*, basophilic leukemia (original magnification ×1500). *Lower*, schematic diagram.

Eosinophilic Leukemia

Marked eosinophilia as such should not be interpreted automatically as eosinophilic leukemia. It is a diagnosis that should be made with extreme caution.[13] The very existence of eosinophilic leukemia is questioned by some investigators and it is considered a variant of chronic granulocytic leukemia by others.[14] Still, a number of cases, including 43, in which autopsy has been performed, have been reported which seem to suggest that eosinophilic leukemia is a distinct entity since any patient with evidence of other diseases which might have caused an eosinophilia were excluded in this study.[13, 14] The following criteria have been proposed for a diagnosis of eosinophilic leukemia: hepatosplenomegaly, lymphadenopathy, and a marked persistent eosinophilia accompanied by anemia and thrombocytopenia. Many patients have exhibited circulating normoblasts. The eosinophils in Griffin's[68] case in 1919, which is purported to be the first case of eosinophilic leukemia described in the literature, were segmented and abnormally large with sparse granulation. His description coincides with two cases that were observed in our laboratory in the past 20 years.

The leukocyte counts in cases of eosinophilic leukemia have ranged between 50,000–200,000/mm^3.[104] Usually greater than 60% of the cells are eosinophilic granulocytes and in over 50% of cases blast forms and promyelocytes have been observed. Some cases have terminated in blastic crisis. Postmortem examination depicting eosinophilic infiltration of organs such as the spleen and lymph nodes have been noted in these cases of eosinophilic leukemia.[104]

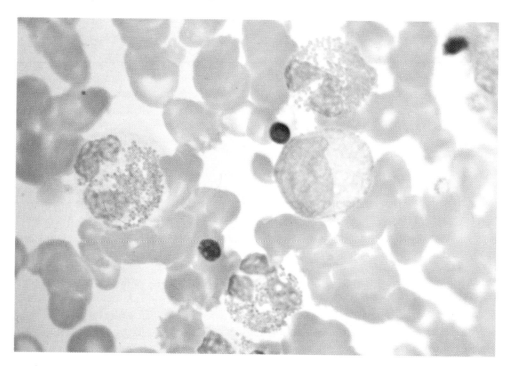

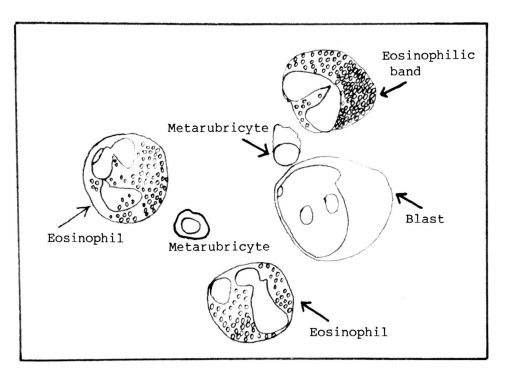

Figure 18.5. *Upper*, eosinophilic leukemia (original magnification ×1050). *Lower*, schematic diagram.

Acute Monocytic Leukemia (Schilling Type)

Acute monocytic leukemia (Schilling or "pure" monocytic type) is characterized by the proliferation of abnormal and immature monocytic cells in the peripheral blood and bone marrow without evidence of a primary abnormality involving myeloid precursors.[183]

The majority of the leukocytes are usually blastic with a secondary predominance of immature monocytes. These acute cases with a blast predominance are often difficult to identify. In one study of 18 cases, only eight were identified by light microscopy.[35, 42] The identification of these immature forms may be enhanced by electron microscopy of cellular ultrastructure[61] and esterase cytochemistry. The two esterase stains[129] most commonly performed to differentiate between monocytoid and granulocytic precursors are: 1) α-naphthyl acetate esterase which stains monocytic cells strongly and granulocytic cells weakly or not at all and 2) naphthol AS-D chloroacetate esterase which stains the granulocytic cells strongly and monocytic cells weakly or not at all. The interpretation of these stains is not without difficulty and in these instances it has been helpful to add fluoride to the staining procedures to inhibit the staining of the monocytic cells but not the granulocytic cells as a further diagnostic aid. However, in some cases of acute monocytic leukemia, the blast cells may possess morphologic criteria that are suggestive of their monocytoid origin such as: irregularity and folding of the nucleus with larger nucleoli than those seen in myeloblasts, more abundant cytoplasm with a greater tendency to vacuolization, and pseudopod formation at the border. The promonocytes or immature monocytes may present in two morphologic forms (see photographs on pages 96 and 97). One form depicts a round nucleus containing one or more creases with a very fine, lightly stained reticular chromatin material. The rounded nuclear formation of this immature monocyte may cause great confusion with the myelocyte stage of the granulocytic series. The second form of immature monocyte has the more characteristic folding of the nucleus with obvious nucleoli and a deeper basophilia to the cytoplasm than is seen in the mature monocyte.

These patients are seen with a moderate to severe normochromic, normocytic anemia which may be due to blood loss, bone marrow infiltration, or accelerated hemolysis. The majority of patients demonstrate a moderate to marked leukocytosis while one-third may have with a leukopenia. Moderate to marked thrombocytopenia is usually present at the time of diagnosis as well.[183]

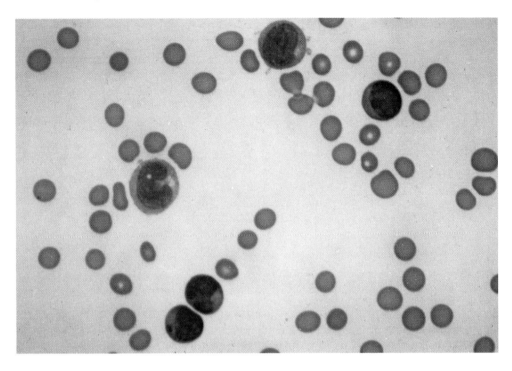

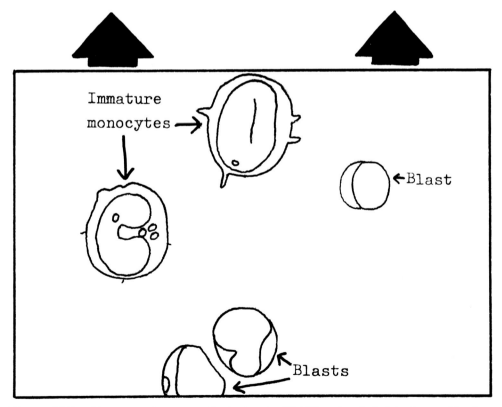

Figure 18.6. *Upper*, acute monocytic leukemia (Schilling type) (original magnification ×600). *Lower*, schematic diagram.

Subacute Monocytic Leukemia

The most characteristic finding in the peripheral blood smear of a patient classified on a morphologic basis as having a subacute monocytic leukemia is the predominance of the promonocyte or immature monocyte with a variable number of blast forms secondarily. The predominance of morphologically definable immature monocytoid cells makes these cases much easier to identify than the morphologically acute blastic form.

In the photograph on page 238, two types of promonocytes or immature monocytes are seen: two smaller, more rounded nuclear forms with creases in the center and a deeper basophilia to the cytoplasm than the mature monocyte and two larger, pale reticular folded or creased nuclear forms with abundant lighter gray-blue cytoplasm with numerous azurophilic granules.

A moderate to severe normochromic, normocytic anemia is present in these cases at the time of diagnosis. A leukocytosis is seen in the majority of patients but leukopenia is not unusual. Thrombocytopenia is usually marked.[183]

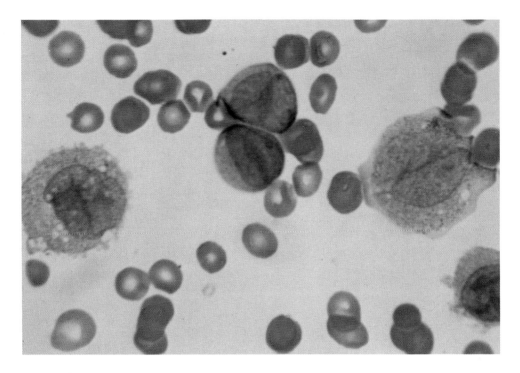

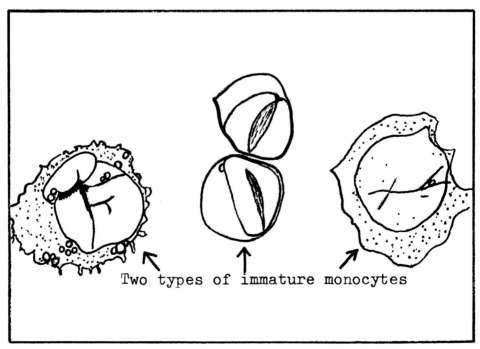

Two types of immature monocytes

Figure 18.7.   *Upper*, subacute monocytic leukemia (original magnification ×1050). *Lower*, schematic diagram.

Myelomonocytic Leukemia (Naegeli Type)

Myelomonocytic leukemia is characterized on the peripheral blood smear by the persistence of immature forms of both the monocytic and granulocytic series.[190] In most cases, the predominant cells seen are myelocytes and immature monocytes. Blast forms are readily found, but promyelocytes are sparsely scattered throughout the slide usually not numbering more than 5% of the cells. Metamyelocytes, band cells, and segmented neutrophils are well represented throughout the slide and often an early eosinophilic or basophilic cell is seen. Frequently, immature cells are encountered which possess both myeloid and monocytoid morphologic features making identification difficult. These cells are classified as "abnormal precursors" indicating that they are blast cells or pro stages of either series but positive identification cannot be made. The term "abnormal precursor" should never be used for a cell more mature than a pro stage of development.

The leukocyte count is elevated in slightly more than half of the patients. Even if the count is normal or low, blast forms are usually seen on the peripheral blood smear.

A normochromic, normocytic anemia is usually found and may be severe. Occasionally nucleated red blood cells may be found in these patients.[184]

Thrombocytopenia is present in most instances, and may be pronounced at diagnosis. Occasionally large bizarre forms are seen.[184]

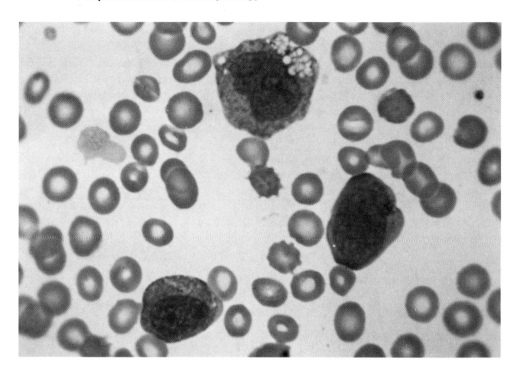

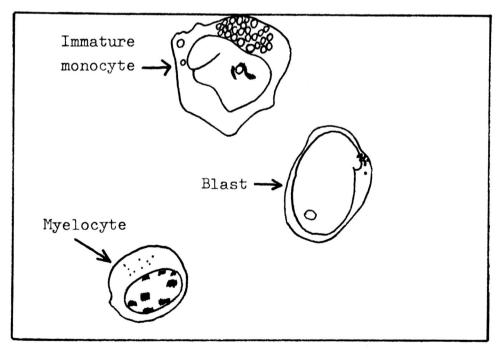

Figure 18.8. *Upper*, myelomonocytic leukemia (Naegeli type) (original magnification ×1050). *Lower*, schematic diagram.

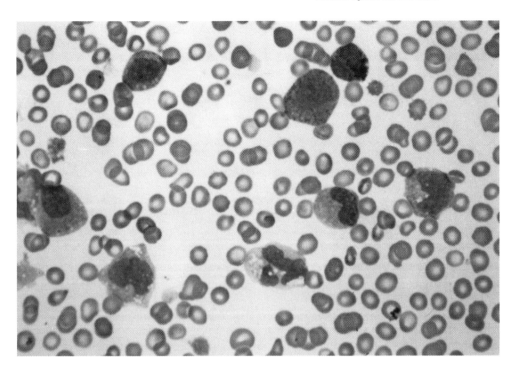

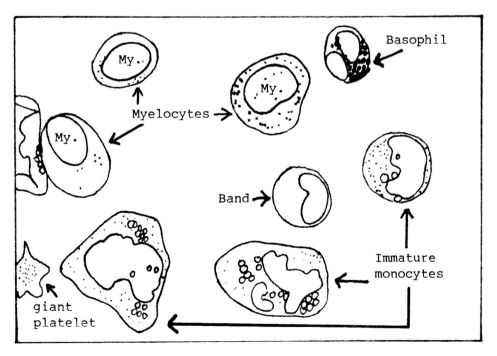

Figure 18.9. *Upper*, myelomonocytic leukemia (Naegeli type) (original magnification ×600). *Lower*, schematic diagram.

Myelofibrosis (Agnogenic Myeloid Metaplasia)

Myelofibrosis (agnogenic myeloid metaplasia) is a myeloproliferative disorder exhibiting abnormal growth of the erythroid, myeloid, monocytoid, and megakaryocytoid cells, variable degrees of fibrosis in the bone marrow, and myeloid metaplasia of the spleen and liver.[183]

The peripheral blood film characteristically reveals the following major abnormalities:
1. Giant platelets (some with abnormal morphology and/or extreme size variation to 8–16 μm in diameter);[144]
2. Immature granulocytic monocytic, and megakaryocytic cells;
3. Nucleated red blood cells (usually less than 5 per 100 leukocytes but occasionally high percentages even outnumbering the leukocytes are found);[104]
4. Moderate to marked anisopoikilocytosis, consisting primarily of teardrop-shaped rbcs and gross ovalocytosis, may be present.[104]

When the peripheral blood film contains numerous teardrop-shaped red blood cells and gross ovalocytosis, the tentative diagnosis of myelofibrosis can be made immediately. In other cases, the diagnosis is more difficult. In general, the differential diagnosis is between chronic granulocytic leukemia and the myelofibrosis-myeloid metaplasia syndrome. The marked poikilocytosis is suggestive but not diagnostic of myelofibrosis. The failure to obtain a specimen which is consistent with a diagnosis of leukemia by marrow aspiration suggests that leukemia is not present, but leukemia cannot be disgarded as a diagnosis because a hypocellular or "dry tap" commonly seen in myelofibrosis may also be seen in leukemia.[104] Needle biopsy of the bone marrow would provide solid evidence for myelofibrosis.

A normochromic, normocytic anemia is present in two-thirds of the patients at the time of diagnosis.[187] It varies from moderate to severe in degree becoming more severe as the disease progresses. Occasionally there is a hemolytic component to the anemia, but the direct Coombs' test is usually negative. Red cell survival is decreased in all patients. Autoimmune hemolytic anemia is found very rarely. Reticulocytosis may be mild (3–5%)[104] or normal values may be found.

Leukocyte counts are variable (1,200–100,000/mm^3), but the majority of the patients show slightly increased counts between 10,000–20,000/mm^3.[51] The leukocytes are mostly mature neutrophils, but some metamyelocytes, myelocytes, and even blast cells can be found. Eosinophils and basophils are increased in many patients.

Thrombocytosis is present in one-third of the cases of myelofibrosis and the platelet morphology is frequently abnormal.[183] Giant platelets and large shreds of megakaryocytic cytoplasm may be seen. Platelet function is also often abnormal. Megakaryoblasts and promegakaryocytes may also be present; in fact, 30/100 leukocytes were seen in one patient here at Yale-New Haven Hospital.

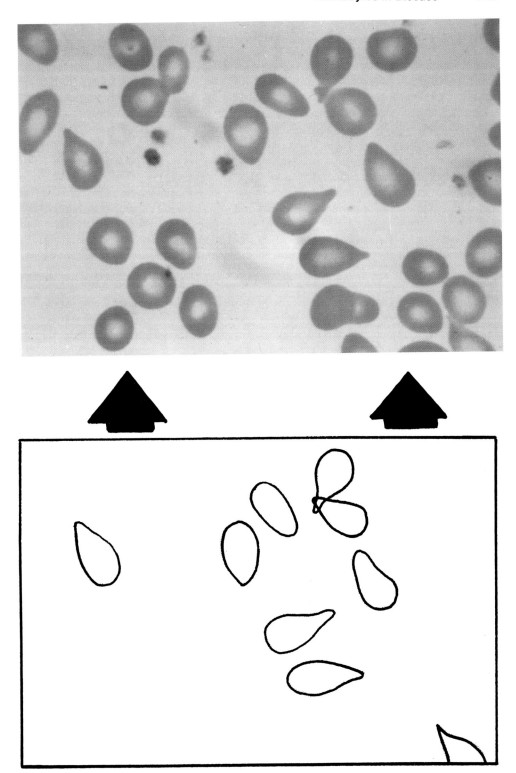

Figure 18.10.   *Upper*, myelofibrosis (agnogenic myeloid metaplasia (original magnification ×1050). *Lower*, schematic diagram. *Note*: only teardrop forms of rbcs outlined.

Acute Lymphocytic Leukemia

The lymphoblast is the predominant cell in the peripheral blood of patients with acute lymphocytic leukemia (ALL). These cells are usually small with a uniformly round or oval nucleus with indistinct homogenous nuclear chromatin which stains intensely blue in comparison to other leukocyte blast forms. The nucleus usually contains poorly defined nucleoli. Generally only one or two nucleoli are grossly visible upon morphologic examination.[183] The blasts contain a scanty, agranular, moderately basophilic cytoplasm. The nuclear:cytoplasmic ratio is usually 4:1 and occasionally 3:1 in these cells. Folded or cleft nuclei may be seen in all forms of ALL, but are most pronounced in lymphosarcoma cell leukemia.[118] The leukocyte count is elevated in slightly more than 50% of patients with ALL and often exceeds 100,000/mm^3 or more.[187] However, the student morphologist should be cautioned that ALL patients may have normal or even low leukocyte counts but blast cells will usually still be evident on the peripheral blood smear in these cases as well. Occasionally a promyelocyte or myelocyte is seen in ALL patients with elevated leukocyte counts and this increases the difficulty of diagnosis.[20] The policy of identifying blast forms by the "company they keep" is not always reliable but generally it is most helpful. A normochromic, normocytic anemia is usually present when the patient is first seen and may be quite severe.[187] There is usually an absolute granulocytopenia and thrombocytopenia. If the peripheral blood and bone marrow smears are exclusively blastic and there are no more mature cellular forms to provide a clue to the identity of the type of leukemia seen, then the term "stem cell leukemia" or "undifferentiated cell leukemia" will be employed.

Histochemical stains may provide important information in these instances, especially the periodic acid stain (PAS) which usually shows large blocks of positively stained glycogen in lymphoblasts and the Oil Red O stain (ORO) which shows 2–4 μ in diameter orange-red neutral fat globules in lymphoblasts. The diagnosis of ALL would be greatly strengthened, if in addition to the positive PAS and ORO stains, a negative Sudan black stain and negative α-naphthyl acetate (nonspecific) esterase stain were found.

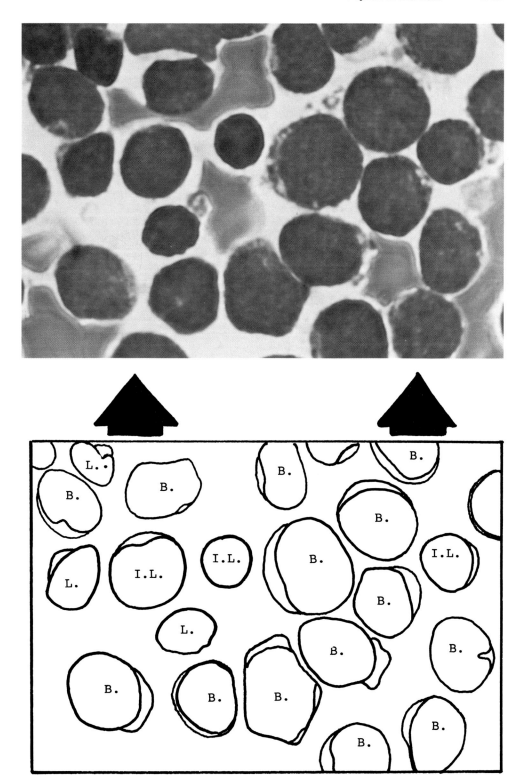

Figure 18.11. *Upper*, acute lymphocytic leukemia (original magnification ×1050). *Lower*, schematic diagram, *B.*, blast cell, *I. L.*, immature lymphocyte, *L.*, lymphocyte, mature.

Chronic Lymphocytic Leukemia

The predominant morphologic characteristic on the peripheral blood smear of a patient with chronic lymphocytic leukemia (CLL) is an absolute and relative increase in the numbers of mature lymphocytes.[187] In mild cases of CLL, the lymphocytes appear almost normal. In the average patient, the lymphocytes appear larger than normal, are more fragile, and easily rupture probably accounting for the moderate to numerous "smudge forms" which are usually observed on the blood film. Occasionally an immature lymphocyte is seen, but it is unusual to observe lymphoblasts in these patients in a 100- or 200-cell differential. The nucleus contains densely clumped, blue-purple chromatin with slightly basophilic nongranular cytoplasm which varies from scanty to abundant in amount in the cells. Occasionally a nucleolus is seen in a few cells.[183]

A normochromic, normocytic anemia is seen in approximately 50% of CLL patients at the time of diagnosis. Occasionally a severe autoimmune hemolytic anemia is seen in these patients. Reticulocytes may be normal or decreased. The leukocyte counts are usually elevated and may exceed 100,000/mm^3 or even higher. Platelet counts may be normal or decreased. Thrombocytopenia is mild when present.[187]

CLL is the most predominant type of leukemia seen in the western countries usually comprising approximately 30% of the cases seen. It is extremely rare in children or persons younger than 30 years of age. The incidence of CLL increases with age and is about twice as frequent in men as it is in women.[184]

The life span of the lymphocytes seen in CLL is quite long and usually coupled to frequent immunologic defects. This has resulted in CLL being described as "accumulative disease of immunologically incompetent lymphocytes."[43] The current concept among hematologists is that CLL is a malignant monoclonal proliferation of Ig-producing B lymphocytes with a block in cellular maturation.

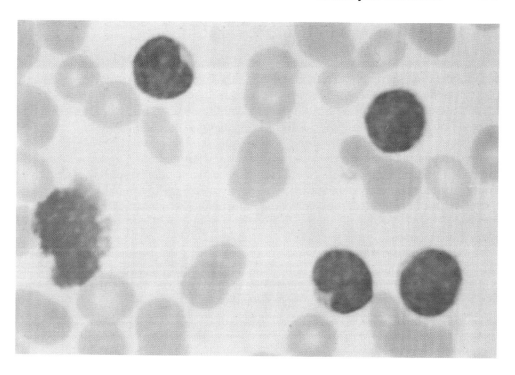

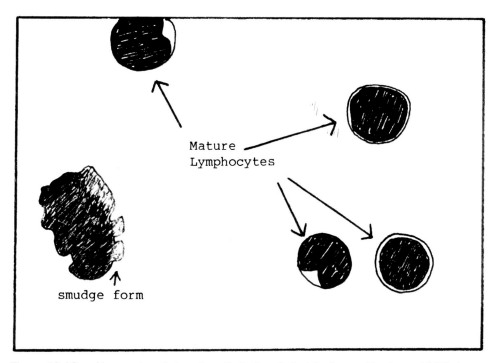

Figure 18.12.   *Upper*, chronic lymphocytic leukemia (original magnification ×1050). *Lower*, schematic diagram.

Cleft Lymphocytes in Lymphosarcoma

Lymphosarcoma is a malignant tumor (lymphoma) which originates and localizes in the lymph nodes, spleen, or extranodal lymphoid tissue. This malignancy involves only one cell line which predominates in tissue sections, namely, small, medium, and large abnormal lymphocytes. In well-differentiated lymphosarcoma, the lymphocytes tend to be small or medium in size and uniform in appearance resembling the normal small lymphocyte. Mitotic figures are rare.[183] These small lymphocytes exhibit dark-staining contracted nuclei, often with clefts in the nucleus and scanty blue cytoplasm.[40] Nucleoli are not prominent. In poorly differentiated lymphosarcoma, the lymphocytes tend to be larger (10–20 μm in diameter) and more variable in size with frequent mitoses.[187] The nucleus is centrally located, round or slightly indented. The nuclear chromatin is evenly distributed and less clumped than in a mature lymphocyte. There is a narrow rim of basophilic cytoplasm.

The diagnosis of lymphosarcoma is suggested by the development of painless, progressive enlargement of one or more lymph nodes or of the spleen in an individual with no evidence of infectious or systemic disease and confirmed upon the performance of a lymph node biopsy to confirm the histopathology of the lesion.[183]

These individuals may develop disseminated disease with blood and bone marrow findings similar to chronic lymphocytic leukemia. However, the cells in lymphosarcoma cell leukemia tend to be larger, more reticulated, and unusually immature. Cleft formation in the nuclei of the abnormal lymphocytes suggests the lymphoma origin of the disease.

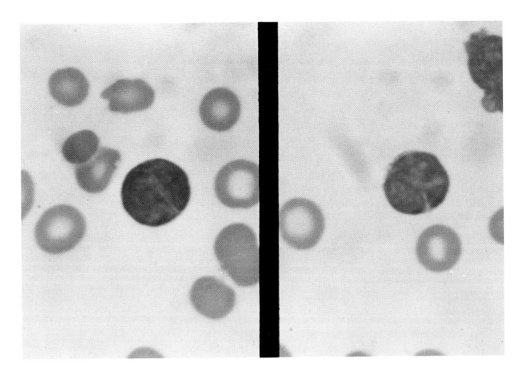

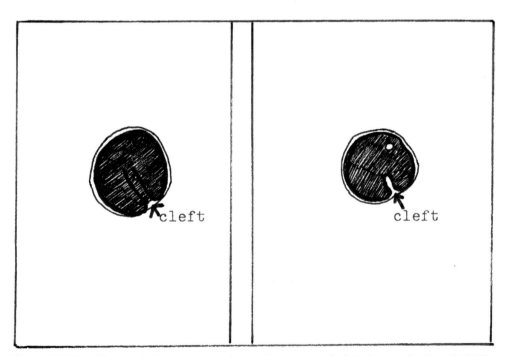

Figure 18.13. *Upper*, cleft lymphocytes in lymphosarcoma (original magnification ×1050). *Lower*, schematic diagram.

Sézary Syndrome (Mycosis Fungoides)

The presence of Sézary cells[159] in the peripheral blood is thought to represent the leukemic phase of mycosis fungoides, a malignant lymphoma, which initially presents with pruritic nonspecific skin lesions resembling psoriasis, eczema, or contact dermatitis, containing the characteristic Sézary cells.[112] Sézary cells are rather large, 15–25 μm in diameter, with the clear blue cytoplasm of a lymphocyte which is fairly abundant.[187] Nuclei are round or oval and commonly exhibit creases or clefts which mimic a monocytoid appearance but contain nuclear chromatin which is densely clumped like a lymphocyte. Nucleoli are not usually seen in Wright's-stained peripheral blood smears. These cells may contain characteristic PAS-positive cytoplasmic vacuoles. Sézary cells respond to phytohemagglutinin (PHA) *in vitro* by acceleration of RNA and initiation of DNA synthesis, and by subsequent mitosis. Since the lymphocyte is the only blood cell to do so, it is concluded that Sézary cells belong to the lymphoid series.[37] The membrane characteristics of Sézary cells are those of "T" lymphocytes whereas the cells in most other lymphomas and CLL have the characteristics of "B" lymphocytes. Sézary cells, because of their abnormal chromosome constitution, are almost certainly neoplastic. In one study of a patient with Sézary's syndrome by Crossen et al,[37] the abnormal lymphocytes predominantly contained a mode of 76 chromosomes and there were two minor modes with 46 and 98 to 100 chromosomes.

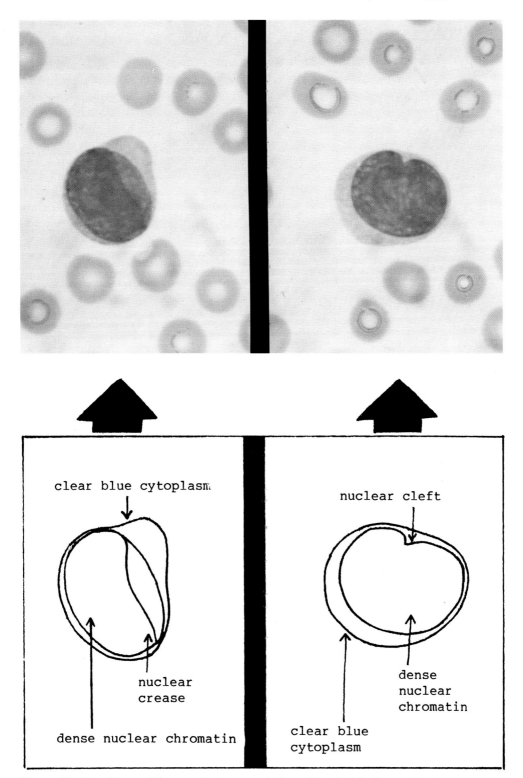

Figure 18.14. *Upper*, Sézary cells in mycosis fungoides (original magnification ×1500). *Lower*, schematic diagram.

Leukemic Reticuloendotheliosis ("Hairy Cell" Leukemia)[58]

1. These abnormal mononuclear cells are called "hairy cells" because of the hair-like projections of cytoplasm which give them a flagellated appearance.[171] They are large (15–30 μm in diameter)[187] with a round or oval nucleus, but occasionally an irregularly folded or segmented one is seen. They have a condensed clumped chromatin pattern resembling lymphocytes in most instances, but some cells have reticular chromatin suggesting reticulum cells. Nucleoli (1–5) are usually small or absent. They possess abundant pale blue or gray-blue cytoplasm. Many cells contain fine or coarse azurophilic granules scattered throughout the cytoplasm.
2. The origin of this abnormal cell is not certain.[155, 171] Recent evidence from histochemical studies and cellular function suggest the "hairy" cell is of lymphocytic origin.[30] This cell lacks phagocytic properties, has surface-bound immunoglobulin and B lymphocyte characteristics, is capable of IgG synthesis with type K and L light chains, and fails to adhere to nylon-like lymphocytes.
3. The specific cytochemical reaction for "hairy" cells is tartrate-resistant acid phosphatase.[187]

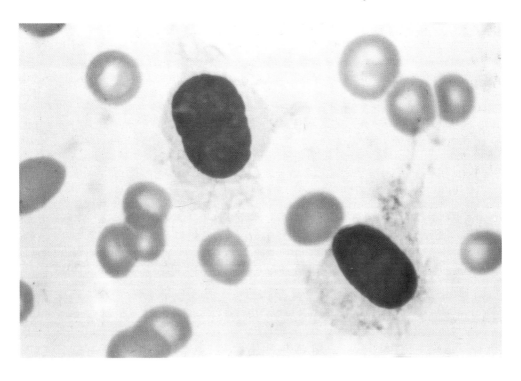

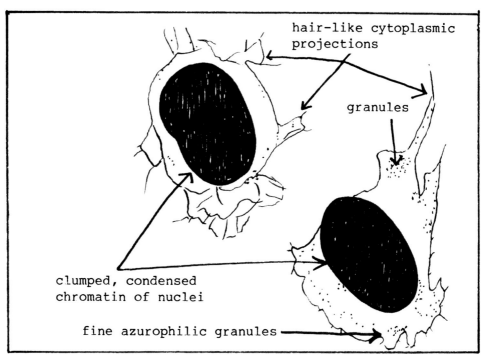

Figure 18.15.   *Upper,* hairy cells in leukemic reticuloendothelioses (original magnification ×1500). *Lower,* schematic diagram.

Infectious Mononucleosis

The most characteristic hematologic finding on the peripheral blood smear of a patient with infectious mononucleosis is the increased numbers of mononuclear cells including normal lymphocytes and monocytes and, in particular, a polymorphic population of atypical lymphocytes. These atypical lymphocytes usually constitute at least 10% and possibly over 20% of the cells in the differential count.[184] They are polymorphic in appearance but generally they are larger than normal lymphocytes with more lobulated or indented nuclear shapes containing dense red-purple chromatin and nucleoli. The cytoplasm may be foamy, vacuolated, or basophilic often with irregular borders that tend to flow around adjacent erythrocytes. Downey and MacKinley, in 1923,[55] classified and described these atypical lymphocytes into three types which are illustrated and described on pages 90–91. A hematologic picture similar to infectious mononucleosis may also be observed in the peripheral blood of patients with cytomegalic mononucleosis (post-transfusion syndrome)[158, 168] and infectious hepatitis[187] although in the latter the atypical lymphocytosis is usually less intense and confined to the preicteric stage.

There is usually a slight or moderate leukocytosis with 60–70% of the patients exhibiting total leukocyte counts between 10,000–20,000/mm³.[59] Of the patients 15% may have total leukocyte counts exceeding 20,000/mm³. The peak values usually occur during the second and third weeks of the disease and may persist for several weeks and even for months in some patients.[88] The leukocytosis is primarily due to the increase in the number of normal and atypical lymphocytes which usually comprise 60%[104, 183] of the differential count and may go as high as 95% in some cases. The platelet count may be normal or slightly decreased in approximately 50% of the patients. Thrombocytopenic purpura is a rare complication and when it does occur it is usually seen in young children. Most cases of infectious mononucleosis are not seen with anemia. However, hemolytic anemia may be a complication in 3% of these patients.[187] In the recovery phase of infectious mononucleosis, an eosinophilia may be noted on the peripheral blood smear. In all patients with this hematologic picture a heterophile antibody test should be done and is usually positive in over 95% of typical cases.[187] In negative heterophile antibody tests with this hematologic picture, an Epstein-Barr virus antibody test should be performed. A positive heterophile result is not diagnostic in the absence of the hematologic and clinical features of infectious mononucleosis.

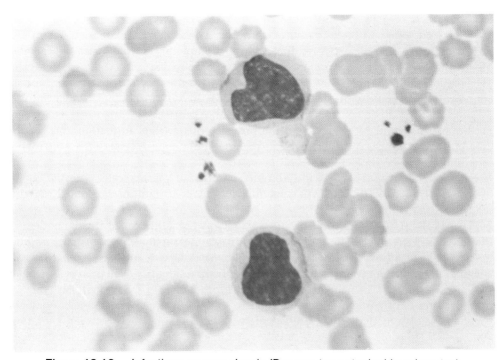

Figure 18.16.   Infectious mononucleosis (Downey-type atypical lymphocytes).

Multiple Myeloma

The most consistent and obvious morphologic abnormality on a peripheral blood smear of a patient with multiple myeloma is the appearance of rouleaux formation of the erythrocytes due to the presence of high levels of abnormal globulins. Rouleaux formation, however, is not specific for multiple myeloma and may be seen in Waldenstrom's macroglobulinemia or cryoglobulinemia. It is difficult for the student morphologist to evaluate true rouleaux formation from the artificial stacking of erythrocytes on a thick smear preparation. It is essential, therefore, that a thin peripheral blood film be made to evaluate rouleaux formation. Examine areas of the blood film in which the erythrocytes appear evenly dispersed or separate and then the characteristic small "stacked coin" effect of three or four erythrocytes will be more apparent.

The presence of rouleaux formation should prompt the morphologist to scan the blood film carefully for the presence of abnormal leukocytes, especially plasma cells and plasmacytoid lymphocytes. If immature or mature plasma cells are seen, in conjunction with rouleaux formation, this would be strong morphologic evidence for a diagnosis of multiple myeloma. On the other hand, if one feels the abnormal leukocytes are the plasmacytoid lymphocytes in the presence of rouleaux formation, one would entertain the diagnosis of Waldenstrom's macroglobulinemia. Plasma cells may represent only 2–5% of the leukocyte differential count in many patients but may be numerous in some patients. If the absolute number of plasma cells exceeds 2,000/mm^3,[184] a diagnosis of plasmacytic leukemia secondary to multiple myeloma may be made.

Plasma cells may contain white or pink vacuoles of γ globulin called Russell bodies.[186] Plasma cells in the chronic form of the disease may appear mature with virtually normal morphology in contrast to neoplastic cells in patients with acute disease which are small, irregular in outline, multinucleated, and very difficult to identify as plasma cells.[183] The peripheral cytoplasm of neoplastic plasma cells producing IgA have reddish tinge or bright red areas of ribosomal protein and are called "flaming" plasma cells. Patients usually develop a moderately severe anemia with hemoglobin levels between 7–12 gm/100 ml.[184-187] In some cases, the anemia may be macrocytic and megaloblastic changes may be evident in the bone marrow. The leukocyte is usually normal but may be decreased and rarely is increased. Platelet counts are usually normal but may be decreased.

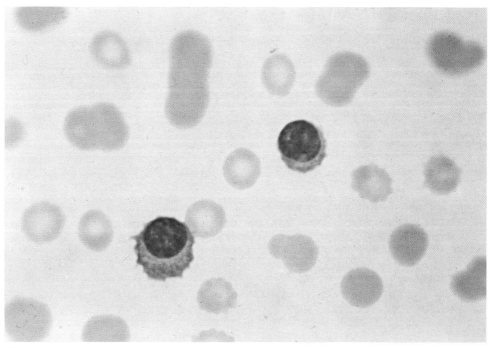

Figure 18.17.   Multiple myeloma (immature plasma cells) (original magnification ×1050).

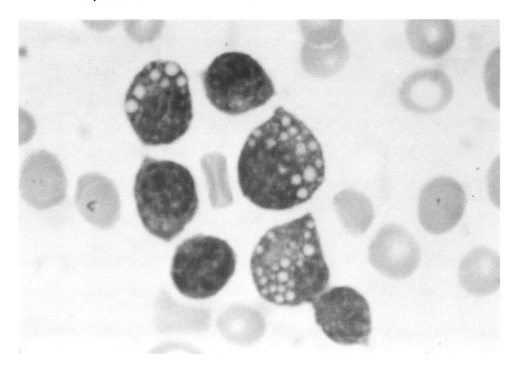

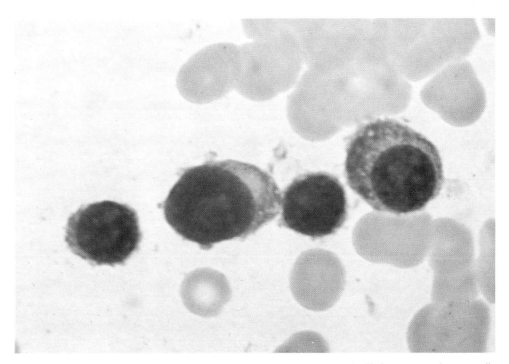

Figure 18.18.   Plasmacytic leukemia (original magnification ×1050). Immature plasma cells depicted; three cells with vacuoles are termed "Mott cells" (*upper*).

MOTT CELLS

1. Plasma cells frequently contain vacuoles even under normal conditions which are small, colorless, and few in number. However, abnormal plasma cells (Mott cells) may show larger and more numerous vacuoles giving a foamy appearance to the cell. If these vacuoles assume a reddish or bluish hue, they are called "Russell bodies" and are associated with increased protein. They are seen in multiple myeloma, plasmacytoma, reactive states, and occasionally seen in some leukemias and lymphomas.[186]
2. Mott cells are referred to as "morular" or "grape" cells by some investigators.[186]

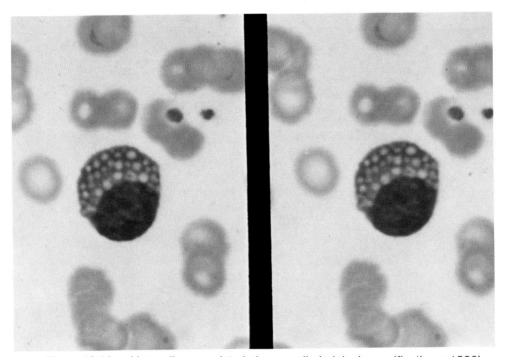

Figure 18.19.   Mott cells: vacuolated plasma cells (original magnification ×1500).

Waldenstrom's Macroglobulinemia

The most prominent morphologic abnormality seen on the peripheral blood smear of patients with Waldenstrom's macroglobulinemia is rouleaux formation. It is due to the presence of high levels of abnormal macroglobulins in the serum. Rouleaux formation is not specific for Waldenstrom's macroglobulinemia but is also seen in multiple myeloma, cryoglobulinemia, etc. It is essential to make a thin peripheral blood film in order to distinguish true rouleaux formation from the overlap of erythrocytes seen in thick smears. Examine areas of the blood film in which the erythrocytes are evenly dispersed and then the characteristic small "stacked coin" effect of three or four erythrocytes will be more obvious. The presence of rouleaux formation should prompt the morphologist to scan the blood film carefully for the presence of abnormal leukocytes. The affected stem cells in this disorder appear to be immature B lymphocytes which retain the capacity to differentiate into the large plasmacytoid lymphocytes and even a few immature plasma cells.[183] In the terminal stages the peripheral blood may contain numerous malignant plasmacytoid lymphocytes. A severe normochromic, normocytic anemia is usually seen in these patients. An increased plasma volume due to hyperviscosity may cause a falsely low hemoglobin value. Erythrophagocytosis has been seen. Leukocyte counts are usually normal but pancytopenia may be seen. Thrombocytopenia may be seen and 50% of these patients may experience bleeding episodes.[136] The Sia test is a useful screening test for the presence of macroglobulins but is not specific and a negative result does not rule out a diagnosis of Waldenstrom's macroglobulinemia. Cryoglobulinemia is seen in 37% of these patients and Bence-Jones protein is seen in 25% of the patients according to one study.[183]

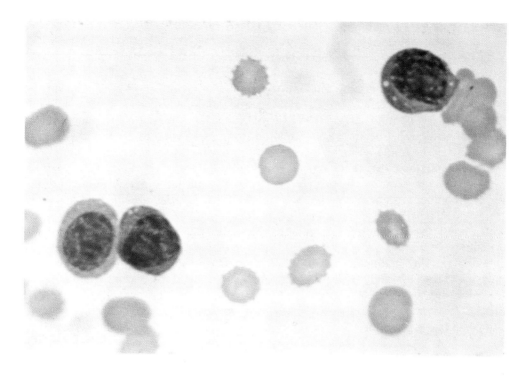

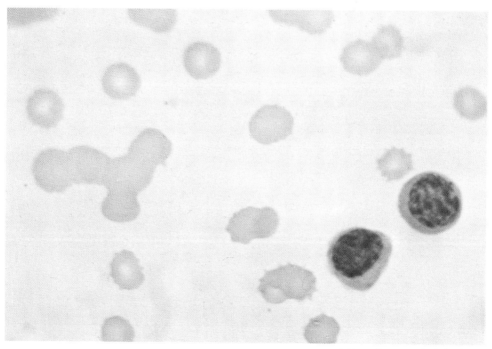

Figure 18.20.   Waldenstrom's macroglobulinemia (plasmacytoid lymphocytes (original magnification ×1050)).

Pelger-Huet Anomaly

1. Pelger-Huet is an autosomal dominant trait characterized by hypolobulation of neutrophils with a coarse, pyknotic condensation of the nuclear chromatin leaving small unstained spaces in the nucleus.[135] Rod-like, dumbbell, and spectacle-like nuclear shapes are common.[90] In heterozygotes with this anomaly 69–93% of the polymorphonuclear leukocytes are bilobed with band counts of 35% or greater not infrequently found.[104] There are very few cells with three lobes (less than 10%) and rarely cells with four lobes.[46] In normal individuals more than 27% polymorphonuclear leukocytes are bilobed and a significant number with three or more lobes can be seen.[167] Homozygotes with Pelger-Huet anomaly are rare and have not been adequately studied.[12] In breeding experiments in rabbits, homozygousity of this anomaly produced cells with round nuclei and no evidence of segmentation and was lethal for these animals.[128] A heterozygous inheritance in humans depicting cells with round nuclei which mimic a homozygous inheritance is known as the "Stodtmeister variant."[137] The acquired form of this anomaly known as pseudo-Pelger-Huet anomaly shows only a few cells with the pyknotic nuclear condensation pattern and three or four lobed polymorphonuclear leukocytes are plentiful.[53] This is most commonly seen in myeloid leukemia with myeloid metaplasia, agranulocytosis, leukemoid reactions, and drug sensitivity.

2. The chief importance of identifying the Pelger-Huet anomaly is to distinguish it from the "shift to the left" that occurs in neutrophilic leukemoid reactions of severe infections especially in patients with gastrointestinal symptoms where the clinical findings coupled with a high band count report from the laboratory mimic acute appendicitis making it difficult for the attending physician to make an accurate diagnosis.

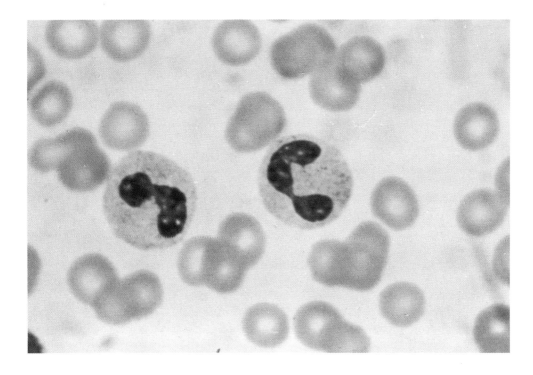

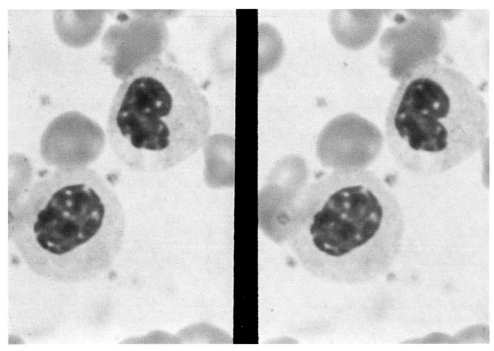

Figure 18.21.   *Upper*, Pelger-Huet anomaly (original magnification ×1050). *Lower*, Stodtmeister variant.

Chediak-Higashi Anomaly

1. Chediak-Higashi anomaly is an autosomal recessive trait characterized clinically by partial ocular and cutaneous albinism and susceptibility to pyogenic infections.[34] Morphologically it is characterized by the presence of large lysosomal inclusions in most granule-containing cells. These abnormal primary granules are the result of fusion during their formation resulting in the large, perhaps defective lysosomes.[84] The specific granules in the cells are normal. Often band and segmented neutrophils contain inclusions resembling Döhle bodies and basophilic granules. The inclusions may also be large, pale pink-orange, or deep red-purple especially in lymphocytes.[187]

2. Chediak-Higashi anomaly is primarily seen in children and young adults although a mild heterozygous form can be seen in middle age.[104]

3. The exact defect is unknown in these patients. The cells exhibit an active oxygen metabolism and phagocytize normally, but the intracellular killing of ingested bacteria is defective and is believed to be due to a failure of postphagocytic degranulation and delivery of the lysomal myeloperoxidase content to the phagocytic vacuole (phagosome).[187]

4. The Chediak-Higashi anomaly has also been observed in the beige mouse, Hereford cattle, Aleutian mink, and killer whales.[183]

5. The Chediak-Higashi inclusions in lymphocytes and monocytes may be very large, measuring up to 3 μm in diameter, and this size range coupled to the pink-orange staining appearance with Romanowsky dyes may cause a resemblance to ingested red cell fragments.[187]

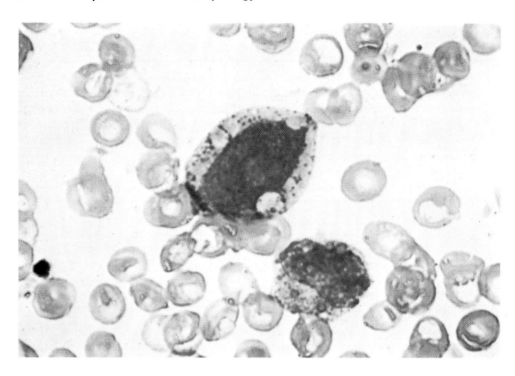

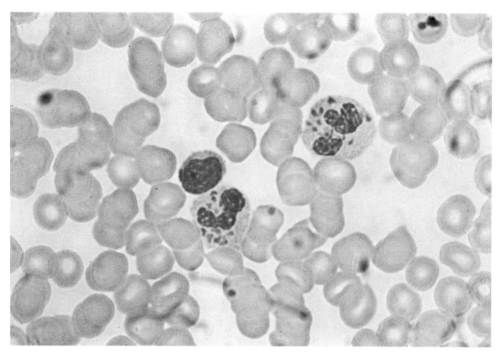

Figure 18.22.   *Upper,* Chediak-Higashi anomaly (original magnification ×1050). *Lower,* (original magnification ×600).

Alder-Reilly Anomaly

1. The Alder-Reilly anomaly is characterized by the presence of numerous large, dark lilac, azurophilic granules in the cytoplasm of neutrophils, eosinophils, basophils, and some monocytes and lymphocytes when the hereditary defect is completely expressed or in only one leukocyte type when it is incompletely expressed.[1, 145] These granules may be easily confused with the granules seen in toxic states due to bacterial infection, drugs, or malignancy.
2. Electron microscopic studies have revealed Alder-Reilly inclusions to be an accumulation of partially degraded mucopolysaccharide within lysosomes.[69]
3. These inclusion bodies are not diagnostic of a particular type of mucopolysaccharidoses but are frequently observed with gargoylism in patients with the various forms of genetic mucopolysaccharidoses including Hurler's syndrome, Hunter's syndrome, etc., which are differentiated on the basis of their particular enzyme deficiency. Alder-Reilly bodies can also occur independently of the genetic mucopolysaccharidoses in apparently healthy individuals as an inherited anomaly (Jordan's anomaly).

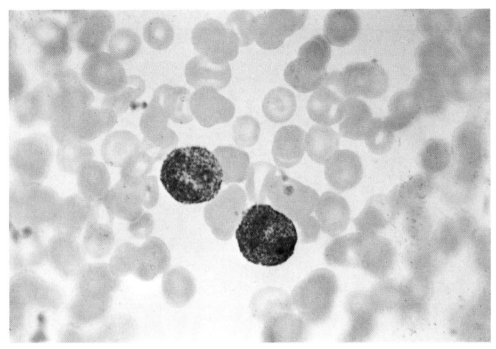

Figure 18.23.   Alder-Reilly anomaly (original magnification ×600).

May-Hegglin Anomaly

1. The May-Hegglin anomaly is a rare autosomal dominant disorder characterized by giant abnormal platelets in the peripheral blood and Döhle inclusion bodies in the neutrophils, eosinophils, basophils, and monocytes.[79, 80, 119]
2. The giant abnormal platelets are the essential feature of the anomaly although morphologically normal platelets may be present as well.[28] More than one-third of the cases are thrombocytopenic. The Döhle bodies consist largely of RNA. They usually occur singly but there may be two in a cell. The Döhle bodies are usually more rounded than those which are seen in toxic states.[187]

Leukemoid Reactions

A leukemoid reaction is characterized by a reactive leukocytosis associated with the appearance of immature forms of one or more cell lines in the peripheral blood which may resemble a form of leukemia but is due to some other cause. The etiology may be severe viral or bacterial infections, metastatic neoplasms, allergies, or drug-induced.[101]

The total leukocytosis is usually greater than 20,000–30,000/mm^3 [133] and is commonly between 50,000–100,000/mm^3.[183] Levels in excess of 100,000/mm^3 are extremely rare. The total leukocyte count may be normal or low in some patients.

Leukemoid reactions secondary to infections are not difficult to determine in most cases because the number of very immature cells (blast forms and pro stages) in acute leukemia is generally out of all proportion to that seen in severe infection in which there is a more orderly increase in intermediate or immature forms. One exception of note is disseminated tuberculosis which can present a myeloblastic-type leukemoid reaction which so mimics leukemia that the nature of the disease may be resolved only at autopsy.[104]

The term "leukemoid reaction" is usually prefaced by the name of the cell line affected, e.g., neutrophilic, eosinophilic, monocytic, or lymphocytic.[183]

Leukemoid reactions may be chronic or acute. The precise incidence of these reactions is uncertain.

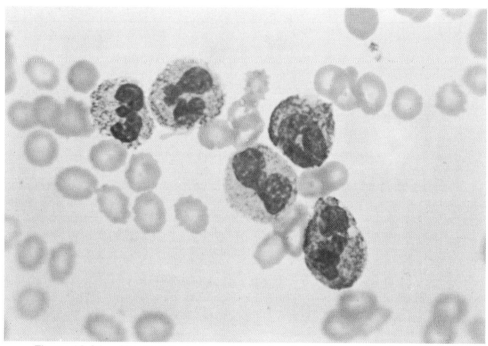

Figure 18.24. Neutrophilic leukemoid reaction (original magnification ×600).

NEUTROPHILIC LEUKOCYTOSIS

Causes:

1. Infections with pyogenic bacteria which may be localized or generalized as in septicemia as well as in mycotic, viral, rickettsial, spirochetal, and parasitic infections.[56, 89]
2. Inflammatory disorders: rheumatic fever, rheumatoid arthritis, vasculitis, myositis, nephritis, colitis, pancreatitis, dermatitis, thyroiditis, etc.[86]
3. Neoplasms: carcinomas, leukemias, lymphomas, especially with widespread metastases.[32, 86]
4. Drugs, hormones, and toxins.[183]
5. Metabolic disorders: eclampsia, azotemia, hepatic necrosis, diabetic acidosis, and gout.[36, 172]
6. Acute hemorrhage.
7. Acute hemolysis.
8. Physiologic stimuli: cold, heat, exercise, pain, cardiac arrhythmias, burns, ovulation, labor, pregnancy, trauma, nausea, vomiting, electric shock, and anoxia.[5, 63, 147]
9. Emotional stimuli: fear, depression, anxiety, joy, rage, elation with anger.[124]

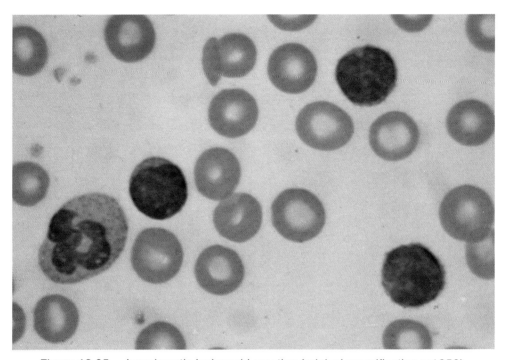

Figure 18.25.   Lymphocytic leukemoid reaction (original magnification ×1050).

LYMPHOCYTIC LEUKOCYTOSIS:

Causes:
1. Acute infections:
   a. Marked lymphocytosis (absolute): pertussis, infectious mononucleosis, acute infectious lymphocytosis, and cytomegalovirus disease.
   b. Moderate lymphocytosis (relative): measles, mumps, brucellosis, typhoid and paratyphoid fevers, tuberculosis, and syphilis.[183]
2. Neoplasms: acute and chronic lymphocytic leukemias, Hodgkin's disease, multiple myeloma, leukemic reticuloendothelioses, giant follicular lymphoma, reticulum cell sarcoma, lymphosarcoma, Sézary's syndrome and carcinoma of the ovary, breast, and stomach.[183]
3. Drug and allergic reactions, autoimmune disease.
4. Metabolic disease: thyrotoxicosis, adrenal insufficiency.[183]

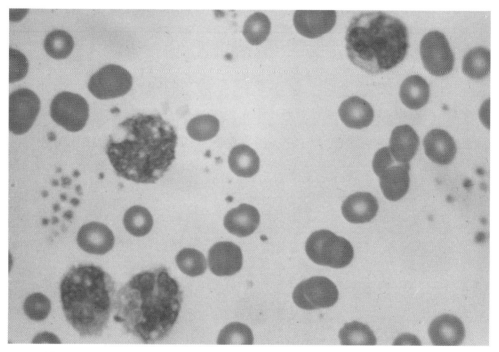

Figure 18.26.   Monocytic leukemoid reaction (original magnification ×600).

MONOCYTIC LEUKOCYTOSIS

Causes:

1. Infections:[6, 41]
    a. Bacterial: tuberculosis, subacute bacterial endocarditis, brucellosis, typhoid fever.
    b. Protozoal: malaria, kala azar, trypanosomiasis.
    c. Rickettsial: Rocky Mountain spotted fever.
2. Neoplasms[115]: leukemia, Hodgkin's disease, leukemic reticuloendothelioses, multiple myeloma, giant follicular lymphoma, reticulum cell sarcoma, and carcinoma of the ovary, breast, and stomach.
3. Convalescence from infections.[83]
4. Recovery from marrow depression due to drug therapy and radiotherapy.
5. Myeloproliferative syndromes: polycythemia vera and myeloid metaplasia.
6. Preleukemia.
7. Collagen diseases: systemic lupus erythematosus, rheumatoid arthritis, periarteritis nodosa.
8. Gastrointestinal disorders.
9. Neutropenia: agranulocytosis of diverse causes.[183]

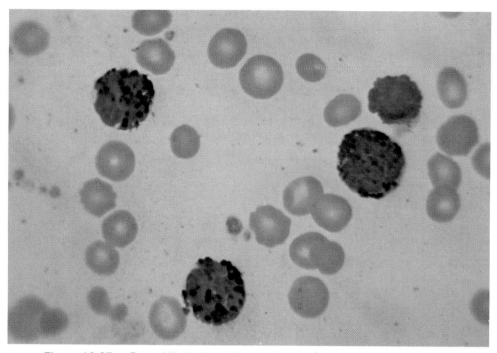

Figure 18.27.   Basophilic leukemoid reaction (original magnification ×600).

BASOPHILIC LEUKOCYTOSIS

Causes:
1. Hypersensitivity reactions: drugs, foods, inhalants, erythroderma, and following injections of foreign proteins.[162]
2. Miscellaneous: myxedema, ulcerative colitis, tuberculosis, diabetes, onset of menses, diurnal (increased at night), postsplenectomy, hemolytic anemia, influenza, hookworm, carcinoma, smallpox, and chicken pox.[22]
3. Hematologic disorders: polycythemia vera, chronic granulocytic leukemia, basophilic leukemia, systemic mast cell leukemia, myeloid metaplasia, postsplenectomy, Hodgkin's disease.

EOSINOPHILIC LEUKOCYTOSIS

Causes:
1. Allergic disorders: bronchial asthma, drug reactions, hay fever, allergic dermatitis, psoriasis, eczema.[52]
2. Parasites: hookworm, tapeworm, echinococcus disease and trichinosis.[52, 105]
3. Skin diseases.[52]
4. Neoplasms: metastatic carcinoma, myelogenous leukemia, eosinophilic leukemia, and Hodgkin's disease.
5. Inherited anomaly.
6. Hypereosinophilic syndromes: eosinophilic leukemia, Loeffler's syndrome, Loeffler's endocarditis, disseminated eosinophilic connective tissue disease, periarteritis nodosa, and eosinophilic granuloma of the bone.[75]
7. Gastrointestinal disorders.

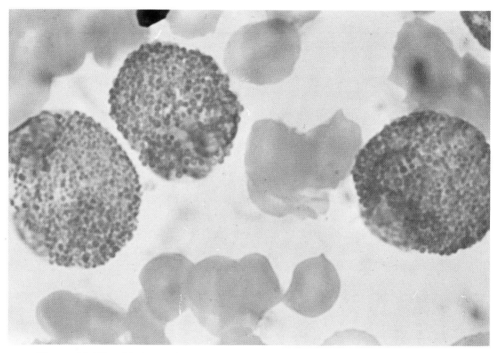

Figure 18.28.   Eosinophilic leukemoid reaction (original magnification ×1500).

Septicemias

The technologist must discipline himself or herself to be on the alert for the presence of organisms on peripheral blood smears for differential cellular examination. If the organisms are intracellular, it is definitive evidence of a bacteremia or septicemia. If the organisms are extracellular, then a source of contamination in the environment must first be ruled out.

It is especially important to detect organisms on the peripheral blood smears of leukemic patients in a relapse state because infection is the most serious threat to their survival. Many of the infections seen in these patients are due to organisms acquired from the hospital environment at a time when host resistance is impaired by severe granulocytopenia.[183]

A buffy coat smear which represents a concentrate of the leukocyte fraction of the peripheral blood specimen is occasionally ordered for differential examination on leukemic patients with markedly reduced leukocytes and even with leukocyte counts greater than 2,000/mm^3 in our laboratory by the hematologists to detect bacteremias sooner in febrile leukemic patients. It is hoped that earlier detection of organisms on buffy coat smears in these febrile leukemic patients will afford them a better chance for survival.

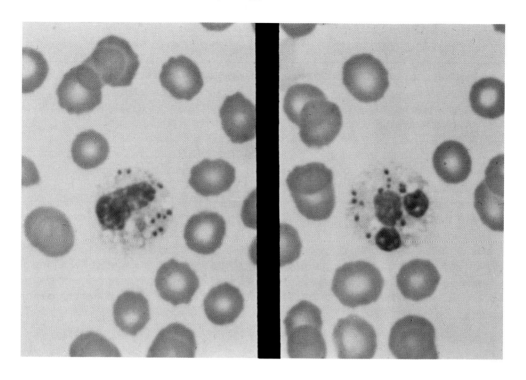

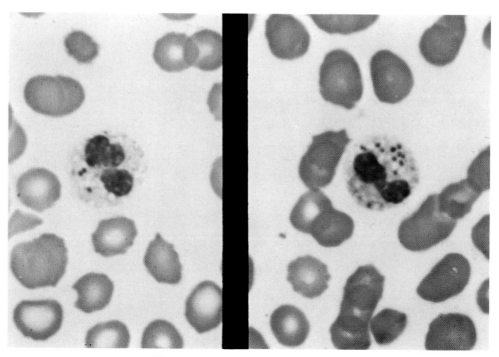

Figure 18.29.   Meningococcemia.

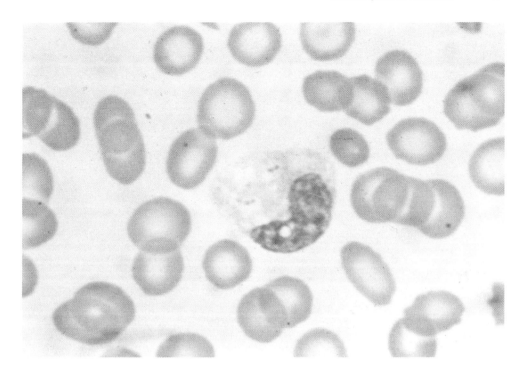

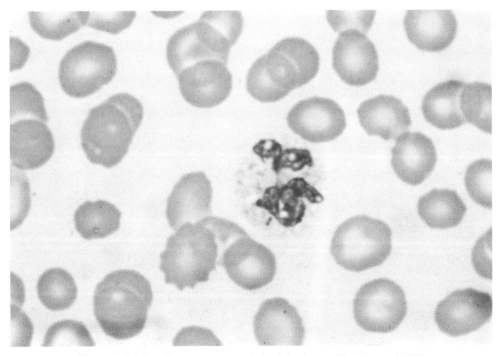

Figure 18.30. Pneumococcemia (original magnification ×1500).

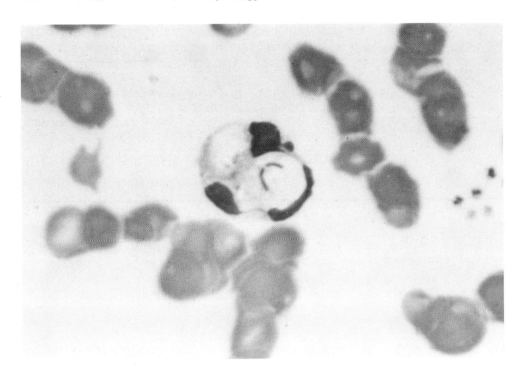

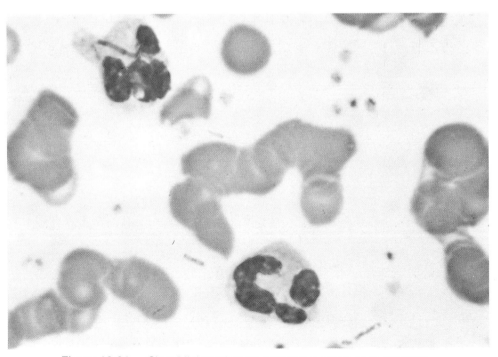

Figure 18.31.   Clostridial septicemia (original magnification ×1500).

Chapter 19

The LE Cell Phenomenon

1. The LE phenomenon is dependent upon an immunocellular reaction requiring three factors simultaneously *in vitro*: a) the LE factor(s) in the γ globulin fraction of serum which act as the nucleolytic agents. These are antinuclear antibodies: anti-DNP, anti-DNA, and a buffer-extractable protein; b) cell nuclei, usually polymorphonuclear leukocytes or lymphocytes, with which the LE factor reacts; and c) phagocytic cells, (usually neutrophils, occasionally monocytes or eosinophils), which engulf the lysed nuclear material.[44]
2. The LE cell is composed usually of a neutrophil with a large pale purple, homogenous, spheroid inclusion (the LE body) in the cytoplasm. The nucleus of the ingesting phagocytic leukocyte, usually the polymorphonuclear leukocyte, is displaced to one side and appears to wrap itself around this ingested material.
3. LE cells cannot be found in smears made from peripheral blood or bone marrow immediately after specimen collection but develop only *in vitro* increasing in numbers up to 1½–2 hours.[40] Therefore, a 2-hour incubation period is ideal for optimum development of these cells.
4. LE cell preparations are best obtained on heparinized blood samples traumatized by exposure to uniformly sized glass beads; or on clotted or defibrinated blood traumatized by mashing clot through a strainer with a mortar and pestle. The traumatization provides extruded nuclei for the antinuclear antibodies to act upon, causing lysis of their nuclear chromatin.
5. LE cells are heavy, due to the fact that they contain two nuclei, that of the ingesting phagocyte and the depolymerized nuclear mass known as the LE body. Therefore, they are usually found in the bottom of the buffy coat layer adjacent to the red cell layer which is important when one is making smears for demonstrating the LE phenomenon.[31]
6. LE cells may contain one or more inclusion bodies. The phagocyte may ingest more than one nucleus or it may represent the segments of the polymorphonuclear leukocyte nucleus.
7. Rosette formation is sometimes seen on LE preparations and represents several neutrophils vying for one inclusion body. Extracellular protein material is also occasionally seen on LE preparations. Extracellular protein material and rosettes, while not specific for LE, are often found in patients who subsequently develop lupus erythematosus and warrant a repeat LE test being performed.
8. LE preparations should be considered positive only if two or more classic LE cells are seen on smear.[31] The presence of rosette formation or extracellular protein material alone does not constitute a positive LE preparation but should be recorded on the patient's requisition for the physician's interpretation.

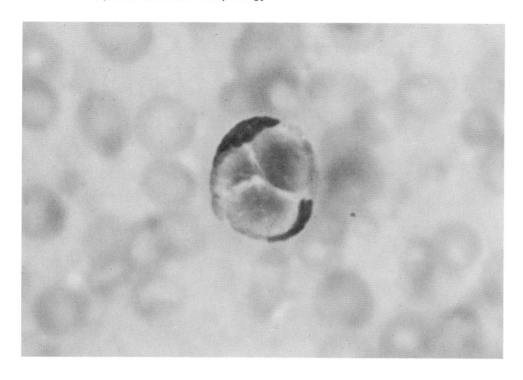

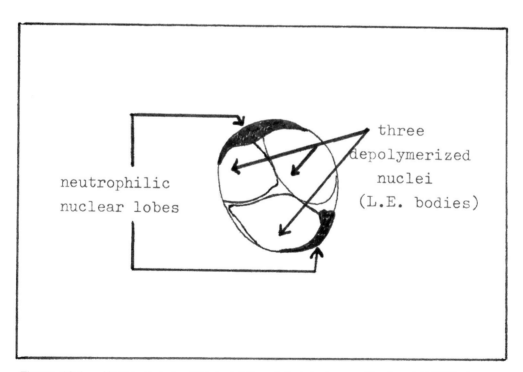

Figure 19.1. *Upper*, true or classical LE cell (original magnification ×1500). *Lower*, schematic diagram.

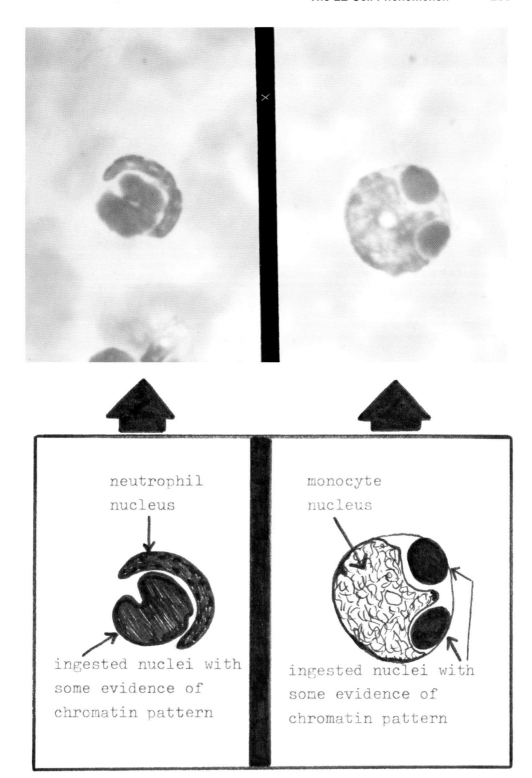

Figure 19.2. *Upper*, neutrophilic tart cell *versus* monocytic tart cell (original magnification ×1500). *Lower*, schematic diagram.

Table 19.1
The True LE Cell versus the "Tart" Cell

True LE Cell	"Tart" Cell
Representative of antinuclear antibodies: DNP, DNA, and buffer-extractable protein[44]	Probably representative of normal nucleophagocytosis[40]
Major morphologic distinction is: *no evidence of intact nuclear chromatin in inclusion body*[31]	Major morphologic distinction is: *chromatin pattern is still evident in inclusion body*
Engesting phagocyte is *usually the polymorphonuclear leukocyte*, occasionally the monocyte or the eosinophil	*Engesting phagocyte* is *usually the monocyte*, occasionally the polymorphonuclear leukocyte or the eosinophil[40]
Inclusion body usually measures 15–18 μ in diameter	Inclusion body smaller, usually 8–10 μ in diameter

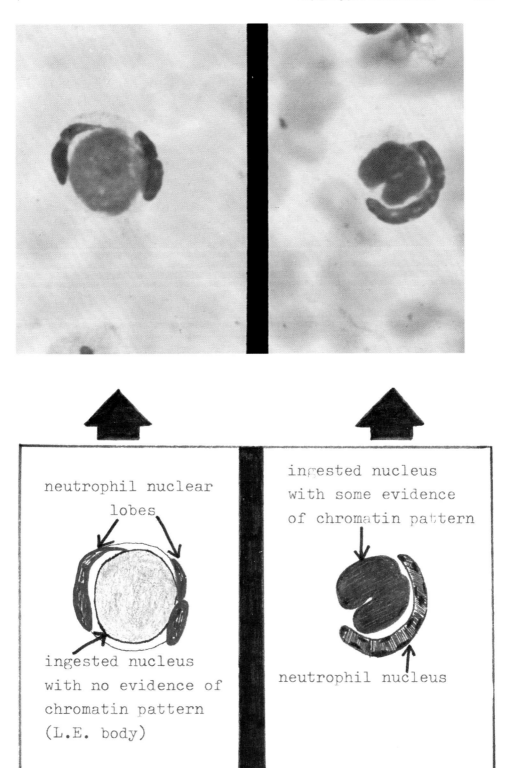

Figure 19.3. *Upper*, true LE cell *versus* tart cell. *Lower*, schematic diagram.

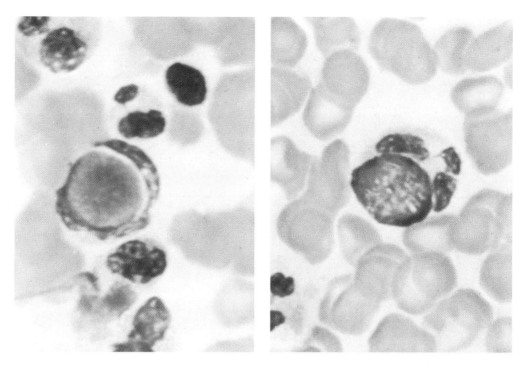

Figure 19.4(left).   True LE cell (original magnification ×1500).
Figure 19.5(right).   Tart cell (original magnification ×1500).

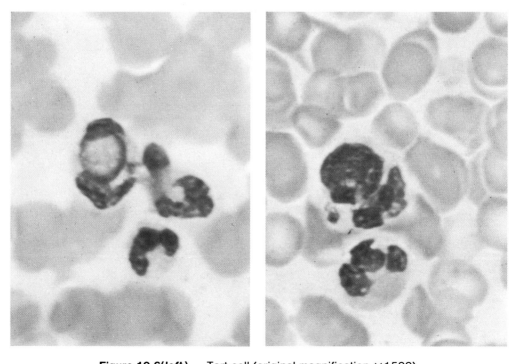

Figure 19.6(left).   Tart cell (original magnification ×1500).
Figure 19.7(right).   Tart cell (original magnification ×1500).

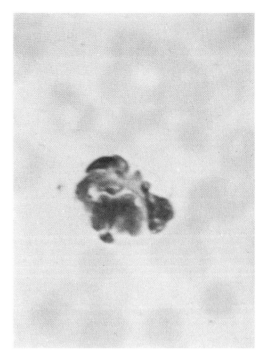
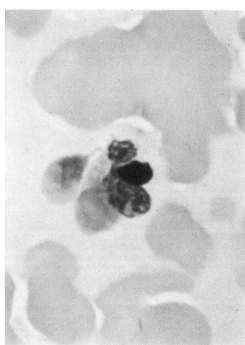

Figure 19.8(*left*). Pre-LE cell (original magnification ×1500).
Figure 19.9(*right*). Pre-LE cell (original magnification ×1500).

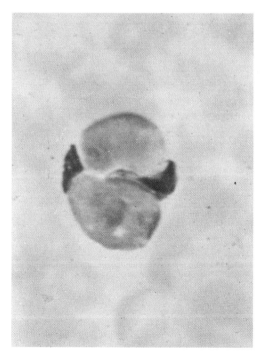
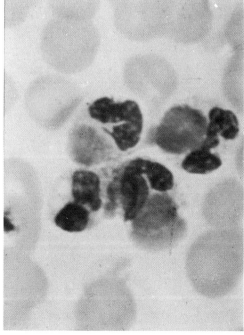

Figure 19.10(*left*). True LE cell (original magnification ×1500).
Figure 19.11(*right*). True LE cell (original magnification ×1500).

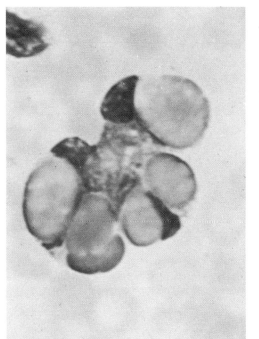 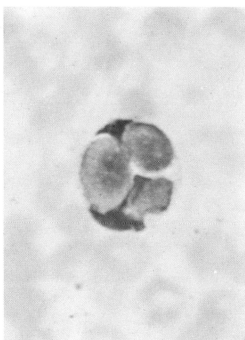

Figure 19.12(left).   True LE cell (original magnification ×1500).
Figure 19.13(right).   True LE cell (original magnification ×1500).

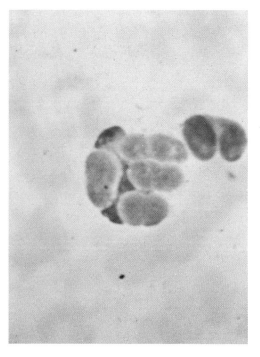 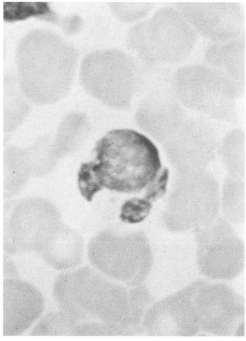

Figure 19.14(left).   True LE cell (original magnification ×1500).
Figure 19.15(right).   Tart cell (original magnification ×1500).

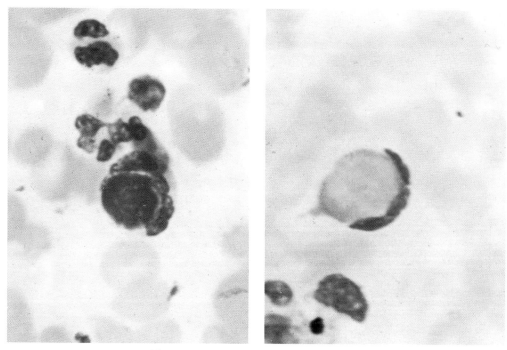

Figure 19.16(*left*). Tart cell (original magnification ×1500).
Figure 19.17(*right*). True LE cell (original magnification ×1500).

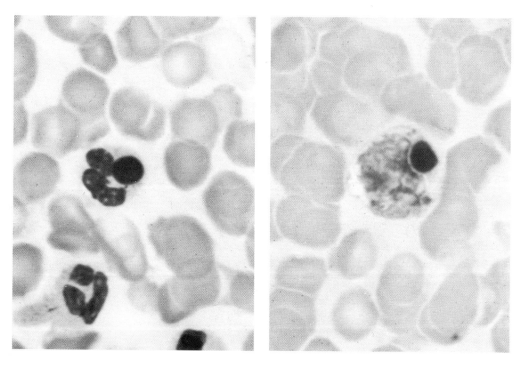

Figure 19.18(*left*). Tart cell (original magnification ×1500).
Figure 19.19(*right*). Tart cell (original magnification ×1500).

Chapter 20

Artefacts in the Peripheral Blood

Various artefacts may appear on peripheral blood smears occasionally. It is important for the morphologist to recognize these artefacts as such, to avoid improper interpretation. If the differential examiner is in doubt, a repeat examination with another specimen, with specific instructions for careful venipuncture and staining techniques, should be performed before a questionable finding is confirmed as an artefact.

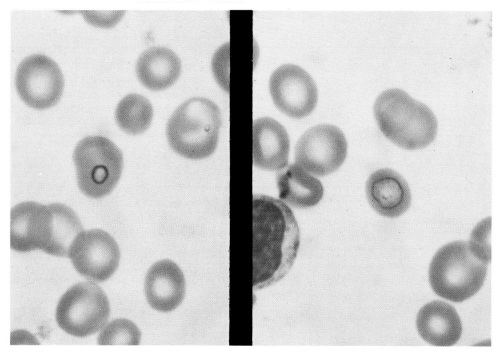

Figure 20.1.   Watermark artefact on red blood cells (original magnification ×1500).

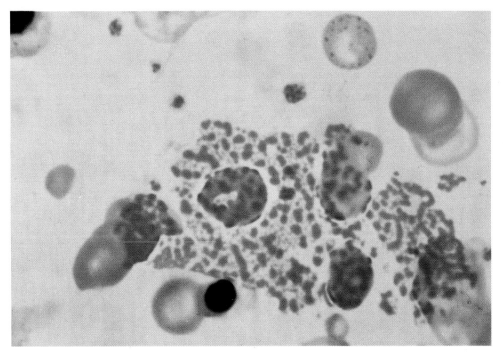

Figure 20.2.   Precipitated stain artefact (original magnification ×1500).

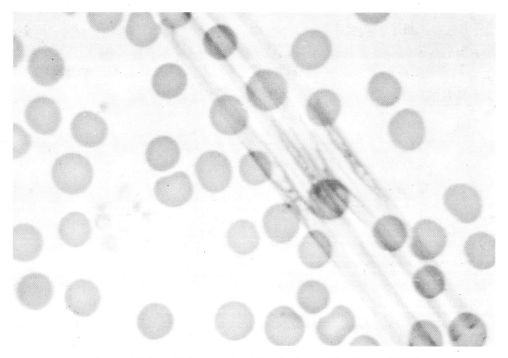

Figure 20.3. Diatom artefact (original magnification ×1500).

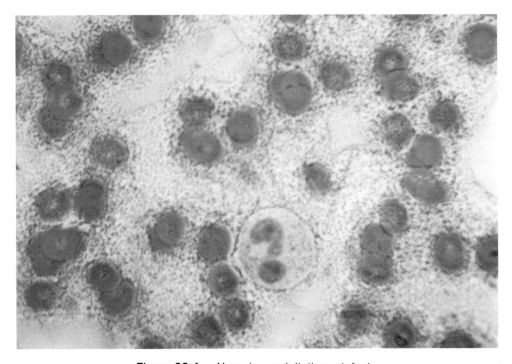

Figure 20.4. Heparin precipitation artefact.

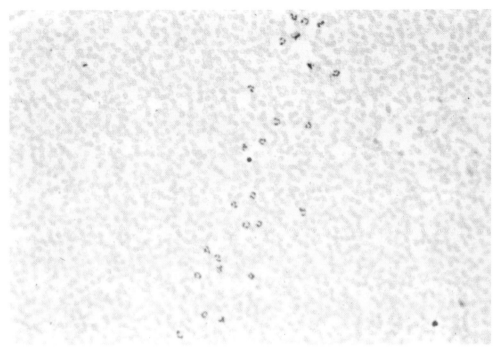

Figure 20.5. Leukocyte clumping artefact (original magnification ×150).

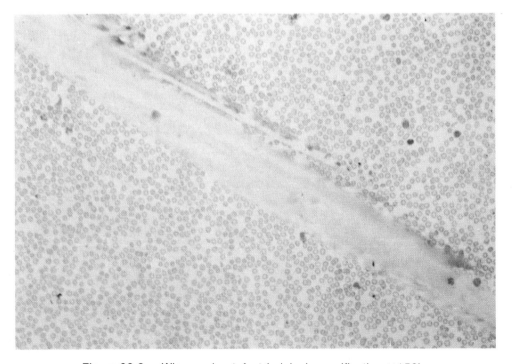

Figure 20.6. Wipe mark artefact (original magnification ×150).

Glossary

Abnormal Precursor: This term is available for use for cells with a 4:1 nuclear:cytoplasmic ratio and immature undifferentiated nuclear chromatin which is believed to be a blast or pro stage but does not fit the morphologic description for a specific cell type.

Absolute Value: This term in this textbook refers to the number of leukocytes per cubic millimeter.

Acanthocyte: This red blood cell is a spherocyte with 2–10 thorny, oblique, projections which was first described in abetalipoproteinemia and is frequently seen in hemolytic anemias.

Achromocyte: A disintegrating, pale-stained red blood cell which assumes a crescent shape (semilunar body).

Acidophilic: Having an affinity for acid dyes; denoting a cell or tissue element that stains with an acid dye.

Affinity: The selective staining of a cellular substance or tissue or the uptake of a dye, chemical, or other substance selectively by a particular tissue.

Agglutination: A reaction in which cells as bacteria or blood cells suspended in a liquid form clumps when the cell suspension is exposed with serum immunized against cells of the same kind and species.

Aggregation: The process of individual units forming a mass or cluster, *e.g.*, platelets.

Agranulocytosis: Acute condition characterized by a severe leukopenia with marked reduction in the number of polymorphonuclear leukocytes (frequently less than 500 granulocytes/mm^3); infected, ulcerative throat lesions are seen as well in the intestinal tract, skin, and other mucous membranes.

Alder-Reilly Inclusions: Red-purple particles of precipitated mucopolysaccharide material in peripheral blood leukocytes, especially the polymorphonuclear cells. The inclusions resemble a coarse toxic granulation.

Anemia: Any condition in which the number of red blood cells/mm^2, the amount of hemoglobin in 100 ml of blood, and the volume of packed red blood cells (Hct) per 100 ml of blood are less than normal. Clinical manifestations include pallor of the skin and mucous membranes, shortness of breath, heart palpitations, and fatigability.

Anisocytosis: Variation in the size of cells that are normally uniform, especially with reference to red blood cells.

Anoxia: The deprivation or deficiency of oxygen in tissue.

Anulocyte: A severely hypochromic red blood cell.

Artefactual: A structure or appearance in a cell or tissue due to death or the use of reagents, and not present during life.

Ataxia: The lack of normal coordination of parts, especially the inability to coordinate voluntary muscular movements.

Atrophy: A wasting away from lack of nourishment or from disuse or from disease, especially pertaining to tissue of an animal or plant.

Atypical Lymphocyte: A benign reactive change in the morphologic appearance of the lymphocyte frequently secondary to viral disease. There is a 2:1 or 1:1 nuclear:cytoplasmic ratio due to an enlarged nucleus with mature chromatin and an increased cytoplasmic complement with increased basophilia and frequently the presence of nucleoli.

Auer Rod: The coalescense of cytoplasmic granules into a peroxidase-positive crystalline rod present in the primitive cells of the myeloid and monocytic series in leukemic states only. Rarely seen in mature neutrophils and monocytes.

Autoimmune: The presence of antibodies produced by an individual against their own tissues.

Azurophilic: Having an affinity for staining with an azure dye especially cytoplasmic granules.

Bacteremia: The presence of viable bacteria in the circulating blood.

Basi-Chromatin: Chromatin material with an affinity for basic dyes.

Basket Cell: A reddish-purple nuclear remnant having a widely spaced thready network appearance with a more condensed central portion which may exhibit a nucleolar remnant.

Basophil: A mature white blood cell whose cytoplasmic granules stain deep blue-purple with basic dyes like methylene blue. Basophils are produced from stem cells in the bone marrow and released into the circulating blood where they are usually less than 2% of the total leukocyte count. The distinct coarse, nonuniformly sized, blue-purple granules characterize the cell which has a deeply staining granular nuclear chromatin pattern and a lobulated nucleus. The precursors in order of increasing maturity are the: 1) myeloblast, 2) promyelocyte, 3) basophilic myelocyte, 4) basophilic metamyelocyte, 5) band basophil. They are increased in chronic myelogenous leukemia and polycthemia vera most frequently.

Basophilia: 1) A condition in which there is more than the usual number of basophilic leukocytes in the circulating blood or an increase in the proportion of parenchymatous basophilic cells in an organ. 2) A condition in which basophilic erythrocytes are found in the circulating blood, as in certain instances of leukemia, advanced anemia, etc.

Basophilic: Having an affinity for basic dyes.

Basophilic Stippling: Blue-purple particles of precipitated ribosomal protein (RNA) seen in toxic states such as metal poisoning, severe bacterial infection, drug exposure, etc.

Bence-Jones Protein: A globulin which represents the light chain of a high molecular weight immune globulin of the plasma. It is associated with multiple myeloma, macroglobulinemia, and malignant lymphoma.

Benign: The mild character of an illness of the nonmalignant character of a neoplasm.

Biconcave: Concave on two sides, especially pertaining to peripheral blood erythrocytes.

Bizarre Red Blood Cell Form: Rare or infrequent red blood cell shapes which do not fit the accepted criteria for frequently seen abnormal red blood cell shapes.

Bleb-Like: A bubble-like protrusion of cytoplasm (*see* Pseudopods).

Blister Cell: A red blood cell with a blister or vacuole devoid of hemoglobin which usually forms near the cell periphery.

Buffy Coat: The layer of leukocyte and platelets lying directing on top of the red blood cell layer seen after sedimentation or centrifugation. It is barely discernible in health but may be several millimeters in height in disease especially leukemic states.

Burr Cell: A normocytic red blood cell with several blunt uniform projections around its periphery.

Cabot Rings: Red-purple single or double rings or "figure eight" loops which can occur in non-nucleated and nucleated erythrocytes. It is uncertain whether they represent remnants of nuclear material, products of cellular degeneration due to toxic substances, remnants of the mitotic spindle, or artefacts.

Cell: The basic unit of structure consisting of a nucleus and cytoplasm of all animals and plants and the physical basis of all life's processes.

Cerebriform: Brain-like folds or convolutions as referred to the nuclear shape of the monocytic series.

Chediak-Higashi Inclusions: Gigantic, peroxidase-positive fused lysosomal deposits seen in the cytoplasm of leukocytes. Inherited as an autosomal recessive trait.

Chromatin: Material within the nucleus which is the chemical carrier of inheritance and determines the nature of "daughter cells."

Circumvents: To surround, *e.g.*, the cytoplasm circumvents the nucleus.

Cleft Lymphocyte: A narrow opening or crack-like fissure at the periphery of the nucleus of small and medium-sized lymphocytes which is frequently associated with lymphosarcoma.

Clone: The colony or group of individual organisms or cells descended by asexual reproduction from a single sexually produced individual.

Coalesces: Grows together into one body.

Coefficient of Variation: The standard deviation (S.D.) expressed as per cent of the mean. It is useful in comparing the standard deviations of quantities which are expressed in different units.

$$C.V. = \frac{S.D.}{\bar{X}} \times 100$$

Condensed: Made more compact or concentrated.

Congenital: Existing at or dating from birth; acquired during development in the uterus and referring to certain mental or physical traits, disease, etc.

Coombs' Test: The direct antiglobulin (Coombs') test detects antibodies attached to the red cell surface whereas the indirect antiglobulin (Coombs') test detects free autoantibodies in the serum.

Crescent Forms: Refers in this text to red blood cells assuming the shape of the moon in its first quarter. Frequently seen in cells containing sickle hemoglobin.

Criteria: Standards or rules for judging or evaluating (plural of criterion).

Cryoglobulinemia: The appearance in the peripheral blood of abnormal plasma proteins characterized by gelling when the plasma or serum is exposed to cooling.

Cytomegalovirus: A herpes virus infecting man and other animals with a special affinity for salivary glands and causing enlargement of cells of various organs and development of characteristic inclusions in the cytoplasm or nucleus. It is species-specific and includes cytomegalic inclusion disease.

Cytoplasm: The substance of the cell exclusive of the nucleus containing various organelles and inclusions within a colloidal protoplasm.

Cytoplasmic Tags: Extensions of peripheral cytoplasm (pseudopod-like).

Dacryocyte: A red blood cell which assumes a teardrop or tail-like formation.

Denaturation: The process of rendering unnatural or to modify (a protein) as by heat, acid, or alkali so as to alter its original properties.

Differentiation: The acquiring or the possession of character or function different from that of the original type referring to cellular maturation in this text.

Dimorphism: Existence in two shapes or forms or outward appearance between individuals of the same species, *e.g.,* both hypochromic and normochromic red blood cells in sideroblastic anemias.

Disseminated: Widely scattered throughout an organ, tissue, or the body (systemic).

Döhle Bodies: Single or multiple round, oval, or filamentous sky-blue inclusions with Romanowsky stains in the cytoplasm of neutrophils especially in immature myeloid cells, monocytes, and lymphocytes.

Drepanocyte: A crescent-shaped red blood cell; usually synonymous with a sickle cell.

Dyscrasia: An old term to indicate disease.

Eccentric: Deviating from the center toward the periphery, referring here to nuclear placement within the cell.

Electrophoresis: The movement of particles (proteins) in an electric field toward one or the other electric pole, anode or cathode.

Elliptocyte: A red blood cell which assumes an elliptical shape; may be an inherited or acquired defect.

Embryo: An organism in the early stages of development. In man the developing organism from conception until approximately the end of the second month; developmental stages from this time to birth are referred to as fetal.

Endoplasmic: Represents the inner or medullary part of the cytoplasm

Endothelial Cell: A flat cell lining blood and lymphatic vessels.

Envelope Forms: (Type I) An erythrocyte which appears folded over upon itself giving a "clam shell" appearance and (Type II) An erythrocyte with its hemoglobin concentrated to one side in the cell giving a flap-like appearance to the cell. They are frequently seen in the hemoglobinopathies and liver disease, especially hemoglobin C disease.

Eosinophil: A mature white blood cell whose cytoplasmic granules stain readily with the coal tar product eosin (acidophilic). They are produced by stem cells in the bone marrow and released into the circulating blood where they represent 0–4% of the total leukocyte count normally. The distinct uniformly sized red-orange granules which cover the cytoplasm characterize this cell which has a dark blue-purple granular nuclear chromatin which is usually segmented into two lobes. The precursors of eosinophils in order of increasing maturity are: 1) myeloblast, 2) promyelocyte, 3) eosinophilic myelocyte, 4) eosinophilic metamyelocyte, 4) band eosinophil. Eosinophils are usually increased in allergies and parasitic infections.

Epithelial Cell: A cell of the membranous tissue covering a free surface or lining a cavity.

Erythrocyte: A mature red blood cell.

Erythrophagocytosis: The phagocytosis of red blood cells or erythrocytes by leukocytes or tissue cells.

Erythropoiesis: The formation of red blood cells.

Erythropoietin: A sialic acid-containing hormonal protein which enhances erythropoiesis by stimulating the formation of rubriblasts and the release of polychromatophilic erythrocytes from the bone marrow. It is secreted by the kidneys and possibly by other tissue. It is present in human plasma and urine.

Erythrostasis: A stoppage or slowing of the normal flow of erythrocytes in any organ or vessel of the body.

Extracorpuscular: Outside of the cell, especially the blood cells. Used to imply an external or environmental cause to cellular disease or defect.

Extramedullary: Outside of or unrelated to any medulla. In hematology usually refers to hematopoiesis outside of the bone marrow in the liver and/or spleen.

Femtoliter: A prefix used in the metric system to signify one-quadrillionth (10^{-15}) of any unit. Used in reporting mean corpuscular volume of erythrocytes.

Ferruginous: Containing deposits of ferric salts in the walls of small blood vessels.

Feulgen Reaction: Employs Schiff reagent which contains carbol fuchsin and sodium metabisulfite in hydrochloric acid to stain deoxyribonucleic acid (DNA).

Filament: Fine, thread-like in structure; often used to describe segmented *versus* non-segmented nuclear forms.

Fragility: Liable to break, burst, or disintegrate as erythrocytes are prone to do when exposed to varying concentrations of hypotonic salt solutions.

Gargoylism: The gargoyle-like facies seen in the genetic mucopolysaccharidoses, such as Alder-Reilly anomaly, Hurler's syndrome, and Hunter's syndrome.

Globin: The protein of hemoglobin.

Glucose 6-Phosphate Dehydrogenase: An erythrocyte enzyme which catalyzes the dehydrogenation (oxidation) of glucose 6-phosphate to 6-phosphogluconolactone in the first step of the hexose monophosphate shunt.

Golgi Apparatus: A membrane-bound compartment in the cell containing enzymes which add more terminal sugar sequences to protein moieties.

Granule: A grain; a granulation; a minute discrete mass usually seen in the cytoplasm of cells.

Hematopoiesis: The formation of blood cells.

Heme: The oxygen-carrying, color-furnishing constituent of hemoglobin composed of protoporphyrin and iron.

Hemoglobin: The red respiratory protein of erythrocytes consisting of approximately 6% heme and 94% globin. Its main function is to transport oxygen to the tissues.

Hemoglobinopathy: A disease or disorder caused by or associated with the presence of qualitative or quantitative defects in hemoglobin in the blood.

Hemoglobinuria: The excretion of hemoglobin in the urine.

Hemolysis: The dissolution of red blood cells with the liberation of hemoglobin.

Hepatosplenomegaly: Enlargement of the liver and spleen.

Hereditary: Transmitted from parent to offspring.

Heterogeneous: Having a different or dissimilar original, *e.g.,* the inheritance of two abnormal hemoglobins; one from each parent.

Heterophile: 1) the neutrophilic leukocyte in man; in some animals the granules vary in size and staining reactions. 2) Pertaining to heterogenetic antigens and related antibody, *e.g.,* parenteral administration of guinea pig kidney emulsion in a rabbit results in antibody that reacts not only with guinea pig antigen but also lyses the red blood cells of sheep.

Heterozygous: Having different allelic genes at one or more paired loci in homologous individuals.

Homogenous: Having a structural similarity because of descent from a common ancestor.

Homozygous: Having identical genes at one or more paired loci in homologous chromosomes.

Howell-Jolly Body: A small spherical body usually no larger than 1 μ in diameter seen in erythrocytes. Pathologcally they are thought to represent a chromosome separated from the mitotic spindle during abnormal mitosis.

Hypersegmentation: An increase in the number of nuclear lobes or segments in blood cells, especially neutrophils in B_{12} or folate deficiencies. In an aged and degenerative neutrophil, there may be 6 or more nuclear lobes.

Hypersensitivity: Abnormally excessive response to a stimulus, *e.g.,* allergy.

Hypersplenism: Greatly increased hemolytic action of the spleen seen in several blood disorders, *e.g.,* chronic neutropenia and thrombocytopenic purpura.

Hyperviscosity: Increased resistance to flow or alteration of shape, by any substance as a result of molecular cohesion.

Hypochromic: Percentage of hemoglobin in the red blood cells is less than normal.

Hyposplenism: Decreased hemolytic action of the spleen seen in several blood disorders.

Hypothesis: A tentative theory or supposition provisionally adopted to explain certain facts and guide in the investigation of other data.

Idiopathic: Of unknown cause or etiology.

Inclusion Body: A characteristic stainable particle in the nucleus or cytoplasm of a cell, tissue, or organ.

Intracorpuscular: Within a cell especially a red blood cell. Used to imply a congenital or hereditary cause to cellular disease or defect.

Intravascular: Within the blood vessels or lymphatics.

Isoimmune: Possess significant titer of specific antibody as a result of antigenic stimulation with material contained on or in the red blood cells of another individual of the same species, *e.g.,* Rh-negative person receiving Rh-positive blood.

Karyorrhexis: A necrotic stage with fragmentation of the nucleus whereby chromatin is distributed irregularly throughout the cytoplasm.

Keratocyte: A term synonymous with burr cells (see Burr cell).

Lamellar: Arranged in thin plates or scales.

Leptocyte: Synonymous with target cells (see Target cell).

Leukemia: Progressive proliferation of abnormal leukocytes found in hematopoietic tissues, other organs, and usually in the blood in increased numbers. Leukemia is classified by the dominant cell type and by duration from onset to death.

Leukemoid Reaction: A moderate or advanced degree of leukocytosis in the circulating blood closely similar or possibly identical to that occurring in various forms of leukemia but not the result of leukemic disease. These reactions are frequently observed as a feature of infectious disease, drug, chemical intoxication or secondary to nonhematopoietic carcinoma.

Leukocytosis: Increase in the number of leukocytes in the circulating blood usually greater than 12×10^9L.

Leukopenia: Reduction below normal in the number of leukocytes in the circulating blood usually below 4.0×10^9L.

Lobe: A rounded projecting part as of a nucleus.

Lymphocyte: A white blood cell formed in lymphoid tissue throughout the body, *e.g.,* lymph nodes, spleen, thymus, tonsils, Peyer's patches, and sometimes the bone marrow. They may be small $(7–9 \, \mu)$ but larger forms are frequent $(10–18 \, \mu)$. The nucleus contains dense homogenous chromatin which stains deep blue-purple. Cytoplasm is scanty, agranular, one-sided, and stains a pale sky-blue. In larger forms, the cytoplasm may be adundant and occasionally contains a few red-violet granules. These cells comprise approximately 25–45% of the total leukocyte count.

Lysosome: Autophagic vacuole; a cytoplasmic, membrane-bound particle $0.5 \, \mu$ or less in diameter; containing hydrolyzing enzymes.

Lysozyme (Muramidase): Hydrolytic enzyme destructive to cell walls of certain bacteria. It is present in tears, other body fluids, egg whites, and some plant tissue.

Macrocyte: A red blood cell $9 \, \mu$ in diameter or larger.

Macrocytosis: The occurrence of increased numbers of large red blood cells in the peripheral blood.

Macroglobulin: Plasma globulin that has an unusually large molecular weight, usually as great as 1,000,000.

Macronormoblast: A large nucleated red blood cell with a normal nuclear and cytoplasmic maturation.

Malignancy: A condition resistant to treatment occurring in severe form, and frequently fatal, *e.g.,* a neoplasm, having the property of uncontrollable growth and dissemination or recurrence after removal.

March Hemoglobinuria: The development of hemoglobinuria following exercise, especially walking or running.

Maturation: The developmental changes that lead to maturity, *e.g.*, stages of cellular division.

May-Hegglin Anomaly: An inherited trait characterized by rounded Döhle-like inclusions in the neutrophils, eosinophils, and monocytes especially and giant abnormal platelets. One-third of these patients exhibit mild thrombocytopenia.

Mean Corpuscular Hemoglobin (MCH): The amount of hemoglobin per red blood cell can be calculated as the mean corpuscular hemoglobin by dividing the amount of hemoglobin in 1,000 ml of blood by the number of red blood cells per cubic millimeter of blood:

$$MCH = \frac{hemoglobin\ in\ grams/1,000\ ml\ blood}{red\ blood\ cell\ count,\ millions/mm^3}$$

It is reported in picograms.

Mean Corpuscular Hemoglobin Concentration (MCHC): A measure of the concentration of hemoglobin in grams per 100 ml of red blood cells. It is calculated by dividing the amount of hemoglobin per 100 ml of blood by the packed cell volume (Hct) expressed as a percentage. This quotient is multiplied by 100 to permit the MCHC to be expressed in a percentage quantity.

$$MCHC = \frac{hemoglobin\ in\ grams\ per\ 100\ ml \times 100}{packed\ cell\ volume\ (Hct),\ percent}$$

Mean Corpuscular Volume (MCV): A measure of the volume of the red blood cells which can be calculated by dividing the number of red blood cells per cubic millimeter of blood by the packed cell volume (Hct) which measures the proportion of blood occupied by the red blood cells expressed as volume rather than percent:

$$MCV = \frac{Volume\ packed\ cells/1,000\ ml\ blood\ (Hct)}{red\ blood\ cell\ count,\ millions/mm^3}$$

It is reported in femtoliters.

Mean: A statistical measurement of central tendency or average derived by adding a set of values and then dividing the sum by the number of values.

Medullary: Related to the medulla or marrow. In hematology the term usually refers to hematopoiesis in the bone marrow.

Megakaryocyte: The immediate platelet precursor cell in the bone marrow. It is a large cell usually measuring 35–160 μ in diameter. The nucleus is usually multilobed. They are normally present in bone marrow but not in the peripheral blood. Platelets are formed by this cell by a pinching off of the cytoplasm.

Megaloblast: Macrocytic erythrocyte precursor due to an abnormal erythropoietic process observed almost exclusively in B_{12} or folate deficiencies.

Megathrombocyte: A giant-sized platelet.

Mesenchyme: A primitive embryonic tissue consisting of mesenchymal cells.

Meshwork: A network of threads. In hematology it is used to describe reticular nuclear chromatin pattern.

Mesoderm: The middle of the three primary germ layers of the embryo; it gives origin to all connective tissue, all body musculature, blood, cardiovascular and lymphatic systems, most of the urogenital system, and the lining of the pericardial, pleural, and peritoneal cavities.

Messenger RNA: It carries the exact nucleoside sequence of the genetically active deoxyribonucleic acid (DNA) to the cytoplasmic areas where protein is made.

Metaplasia: The abnormal transformation of an adult, fully differentiated tissue of one kind into a differentiated tissue of another kind.

Metastatic: The presence of neoplasms in parts of the body remote from the origin of the primary tumor.

Micelle: An elongated sub(light)microscopic particle detected by hydrogels; of supramolecular character and crystalline structure.

Microangiopathic: Refers to pathologic lesions affecting the capillaries.

Microcyte: A red blood cell which is less than 6 μ in diameter; usually 3–5 μ in diameter.

Microcytosis: The occurrence of increased numbers of smaller than normal red blood cells in the peripheral blood.

Microspherocyte: A smaller and more globular spherocyte than usual seen in hemolytic icterus.

Microvasculature: The system of small blood vessels.

Mitochondria: Organelles of cell cytoplasm which are the principal energy source of the cell and contain the cytochrome enzymes of terminal electron transport and the enzymes of the citric acid cycle, fatty acid oxidation, and oxidative phosphorylation.

Mitosis: The process of cellular division or reproduction consisting of a sequence of nuclear modifications (prophase, metaphase, anaphase, and telophase) that result in the formation of two daughter cells with exactly the same chromosome and deoxyribonucleic acid (DNA) content as that of the original or mother cell.

Monocyte: A white blood cell which normally constitutes 3–10% of the total leukocyte count in the peripheral blood; in addition, they are normally found in lymph nodes, spleen, bone marrow, and loose connective tissue. They have a central cerebriform or folded nucleus with pale-staining reticular chromatin. The abundant cytoplasm stains gray-blue and contains numerous fine red lysosomal granules. The cytoplasm is frequently vacuolated and the border often shows "bleb-like" protrusions.

Morphology: The science of external structure and form without regard to function.

Mucopolysaccharidosis: A group of diseases which have in common a disorder in the metabolism of mucopolysaccharides which comprise most of the ground substance of connective tissue.

Multipotential: Used to describe a stem cell that has the capacity or potential to develop into more than one cell line in this text.

Mutant: An individual possessing one or more genes that have undergone a change in character that is perpetuated in subsequent divisions of the cell in which it occurs.

Myelofibrosis: Generalized fibrosis of the bone marrow associated with myeloid metaplasia of the spleen and other organs, leukoerythroblastic anemia, and thrombocytopenia although the bone marrow often contains many megakaryocytes.

Necrobiosis: Physiologic or normal death of cells or tissue as a result of changes associated with development, aging, or use ("wear and tear" degeneration).

Necrosis: The pathologic death of one or more cells or of a portion of tissue or organ, resulting from irreversible damage.

Neoplastic: Characterized by a neoplasm (a new growth; an abnormal tissue that grows by cellular proliferation more rapidly than normal and continues to grow after the stimulus that initiated the growth ceases to exist).

Neutropenia: The presence of abnormally small numbers of neutrophils in the circulating blood.

Neutrophil: A mature white blood cell produced from stem cells in the bone marrow and, in some pathologic conditions, extramedullary sites such as the spleen and/or liver. They are released into the circulating blood where they represent 54–65% of the total leukocyte count. With Romanowsky dyes: 1) the nucleus stains dark blue-purple and is lobulated (normally 2–5 lobes), connected by thin (less than 1 μ in diameter) strands of chromatin with coarsely granular chromatin within the lobes; 2) pale pink cytoplasm with numerous fine lilac (violet-pink) granules (*i.e.,* not acidophilic or basophilic as in eosinophils or basophils). The precursors of neutrophils in order of increasing maturity are: 1) myeloblast, 2) promyelocyte, 3) myelocyte, 4) metamyelocyte, 5) band neutrophil (nonsegmented or "stab" forms). The term "neutrophil" usually indicates only the mature form even though neutrophilic granules are seen in three of the immature forms of its series. In the younger forms the term "neutrophilic" precedes the stage name such as myelocyte, *e.g.,* neutrophilic myelocyte. The term "neutrophil" is also noted for cells or tissues that have no special affinity for acid or basic dyes, *i.e.,* the cytoplasm stains equally with either type of dye. They are usually increased in toxic states, especially bacterial infections.

Neutrophilia: An increase in the number of neutrophils in the circulating blood (or in tissue or both).

Nocturnal: Pertaining to the hours of darkness (night).

Normoblast: A nucleated red blood cell; the immediate prescursor of a normal erythrocyte in man. Its four stages of development are: 1) pronormoblast, 2) basophilic normoblast, 3) polychromatophilic normoblast, 4) orthochromic normoblast.

Normochromic: The amount of hemoglobin in the red blood cell is normal.

Normocytic: Pertains to red blood cells being of normal size (6–8 μ in diameter).

Nucleolus: A small spherical mass of basophilic material within the nuclear chromatin. It is usually single, but 2–5 nucleoli may be seen. Usually prominent in early cell stages (blast and pro stage).

Nucleus: A round, oval, or cerebriform body found in cells which is the essential agent in growth, metabolism, reproduction, and transmission of cellular characteristics.

Oblique: Neither perpendicular nor horizontal; slanting; inclined.

Opaque: Not reflecting or giving out light.

Ovalocyte: An oval or elliptical (elliptocyte) red blood cell.

Oxychromatin: That portion of chromatin which has an affinity for acidic dyes.

Pancytopenia: Reduction in the number of erythrocytes, leukocytes, and platelets in the peripheral blood.

Panoptic: All revealing; denoting the effect of multiple or differential staining.

Pappenheimer Bodies: Small aggregates of irregular basophilic inclusions in red blood cells on Wright's-stained smears which are believed to be iron particles and must be confirmed as such by the Prussian blue reaction.

Parachromatin: Unstained or lightly stained portions of the nucleus adjacent to chromatin material.

Paroxysmal: Refers to occurring in paroxysms (sharp spasm) or sudden onset of a symptom or disease, especially one with recurrent manifestations, *e.g.,* paroxysmal nocturnal hemoglobinuria and paroxysmal cold hemoglobinuria.

Pathogenesis: The mode of origin or development of any disease or marked process.

Pelger-Huet Anomaly: An autosomal dominant trait characterized by hypolobulation of neutrophils with a coarse pyknotic condensation of nuclear chromatin leaving small unstained spaces in the nucleus.

Perinuclear: Surrounding a nucleus.

Pernicious: Destructive; indicating a disease of severe character and usually fatal without specific treatment, *e.g.,* pernicious anemia, the original term for vitamin B_{12} deficiency before specific therapy was found.

Phagocyte: Carrier cell; scavenger cell; a cell which possesses the property of ingesting bacteria, foreign particles, and other cells. Phagocytes are usually divided into two classes: 1) microphages (polymorphonuclear leukocytes), which ingest chiefly bacteria and 2) Macrophages (histiocytes and monocytes), which are largely scavengers ingesting dead tissue and degenerated cells.

Phytohemagglutinin: A plant lectin that agglutinates red blood cells.

Picogram: A prefix used in the metric system to signify 10^{-12}.

Plasma Cell: A white blood cell infrequently seen in the bone marrow of healthy individuals which has an eccentrically placed nucleus containing coarsely granular blue-purple chromatin. Adjacent to the nucleus is a perinuclear clear zone. The one-sided cytoplasm is basophilic and often contains small white vacuoles near the periphery. These cells are not usually seen in the peripheral blood except in viral disease, immunological reactions, and multiple myeloma patients.

Platelet Satellitosis: Platelets surrounding the periphery of a neutrophil.

Pluripotential: Having the capacity to develop more than one cell line, as used in this text.

Poikilocytosis: The presence of abnormal shapes of red blood cells in the peripheral blood.

Polychromatophilic (Polychromasia): A tendency of red blood cells to stain with basic and acid dyes giving a diffuse gray-blue appearance to the cells.

Polycythemia: An increase above normal in the number of erythrocytes in the peripheral blood.

Polymorphic: Occurring in more than one morphologic form.

Prosthesis: A fabricated substitute for a missing part of the body, *e.g.,* a heart valve, tooth, eye, limb, etc.

Protoporphyrin: The substituted porphyrin that, with iron, forms the heme of hemoglobin and the prosthetic groups of myoglobin, catalase, cytochromes, etc.

Pseudopods: A temporary cytoplasmic process put forth for locomotion or for ingesting food.

Punctate: Marked with dots, *e.g.,* the red blood cell with a toxic precipitation of ribosomal protein (RNA) (basophilic stippling).

Purpura: A condition characterized by small red-purple hemorrhages into the skin (petechiae) and mucous membranes related to decreased or dysfunctional platelets or platelet antibodies.

Pyknotic: Pertaining to a condensation and reduction in the size of a cell or its nucleus, usually associated with hyperchromatosis (intense pigmentation or staining).

Pyogenic: Pertaining to the formation of pus, *e.g.,* pyogenic infection.

Qualitative: Pertaining to quality (merit)

Quantitative: Pertaining to quantity (number).

Ratio: Proportion; an expression of the relation of one quanity to another.

Refractory: Obstinate, not responsive to therapy.

Rgenerative: Pertaining to reproduction or reconstitution of a lost or injured part.

Relative Value: This term is applied in this text to the percentage of cells found in a 100-cell differential leukocyte count of a peripheral blood smear.

Remnant: A small fragment, *e.g.,* as of a cell or part of a cell.

Reticular: Refers to a chromatin pattern which consists of a fine network of threads seen in the monocytic series.

Reticulocyte: A young red blood cell with a network of precipitated basophilic substance (RNA) occuring during the process of active blood regeneration posthemorrhagic or posthemolytic.

Reticulum: A fine network formed by cells, or formed by certain structures within cells or of connective tissue fibers between cells.

Ribosomal: Pertaining to granules of ribonucleoprotein.

Rouleaux: A "stacked coin" effect of red blood cells due to an abnormal protein coating on the cell's surface; seen in multiple myeloma and Waldenstrom's macroglobulinemia.

Schistocyte (Schizocyte): A fragmented red blood cell.

Semilunar Body: See Achromocyte.

Septicemia: Septic intoxication caused by the presence and multiplication of microorganisms in the circulating blood.

Sequestration: To remove or separate, *e.g.,* the removal by the spleen of deformed or aged red blood cells from the circulating blood.

Shift to the Left: Indicates an increase in the number of cells with only one lobe or very few lobes in the nucleus or the more immature leukocyte forms, *e.g.,* high nonsegmented neutrophil count in severe infection.

Shift to the Right: Represents an increase in the number of nuclear lobes above normal, *e.g.,* hypersegmented neutrophils seen in B_{12} or folate deficiency.

Sideroblast: A nucleated red blood cell containing iron particles confirmed by a specific iron stain such as the Prussian blue reaction.

Siderocyte: A non-nucleated red blood cell containing iron particles confirmed by a specific iron stain such as the Prussican blue reaction.

Smudge Form: A reddish-purple nuclear remnant with a compact arrangement of material occasionally exhibiting one or two indistinct nucleolar areas.

Spectrin: A large molecular weight protein found on the inner surface of the red blood cell membrane.

Spherocyte: A globular red blood cell lacking central pallor and usually microcytic in diameter, but with an increased cell thickness.

Splenectomy: The removal of the spleen.

Splenomegaly: Enlargement of the spleen seen in several blood disorders.

Spur Cell: A synonym for acanthocyte.

Spurious: Illegitimate, false.

Standard Deviation: The standard deviation (S.D.) is a measure of the variability about the mean. The average or mean ($\bar{X}$) is defined as the sum of all of the observations (SX) divided by the number of observations (N). One standard deviation on each side of the mean (±1 S.D.) is defined as that value which takes in approximately 68% of the determinations. Two standard deviations on each side of the mean (±2 S.D.) includes about 95% of the determinations. The standard deviation is expressed in the same units as the quantity measured:

$$\text{S.D.} = \sqrt{\frac{S\,(X - \bar{X})^2}{(N - 1)}}$$

Steatorrhea: The passage of fat in large amounts in the feces.

Stem Cell: A cell in which the progeny (daughter cells) of cellular division are identical in appearance and potential to that of the mother cell.

Stomatocyte: A red blood cell with slit-like hypochromia.

Tailed Red Blood Cell: See Dacryocyte.

Target Cell: A thin red blood cell of greater than normal diameter which exhibits a centrally placed pink cytoplasmic area with a surrounding ring of pallor which is in turn surrounded by a circle of pink cytoplasm.

Teardrop Red Blood Cell: See Dacryocyte.

Tetragonal: Possessing four sides; quadruple.

Thrombocyte: A platelet.

Thrombocytopenia: A reduction in the number of platelets in the circulating blood.

Thrombocytosis: An increase in the number of platelets in the circulating blood.

Thrombus: A clot in a blood vessel or in one of the cavities of the heart formed during life from blood constituents; it may be occlusive or attached to the vessel of the heart wall without obstructing the lumen.

Toxic Granulation: Dark, basophilic granulation in the cytoplasm of late stage myeloid cells and monocytes usually which varies from fine to coarse in consistency and from few to numerous in number. Believed to represent the toxic precipitation of ribosomal protein (RNA).

Transferrin: Plasma globulin which transports iron in the circulating blood.

Truncate: To round off as with figures or numbers.

Unidentified Mononuclear Cell: A mononuclear cell which does not fit the classic morphologic description of a specific cell type.

Unidentified Polynuclear Cell: A polynuclear cell which does not fit the classic morphologic description of a specific cell type.

Vacuoles: Minute empty spaces in the substance of a cell, sometimes degenerative in character, sometimes surrounding an engulfed foreign body and serving as a temporary cell stomach for the digestion of a body.

Variant: That which is diversified or variable; a tendency to alter or change, not conform to or to differ from the type.

Viremia: The presence of viruses in the circulating blood.

References

1. Alder, A.: Über konstitutionell bedingte Granulations veranderungen der Leukocyten. *Dtsch. Arch. Klin. Med.* 183:372, 1939.
2. Allen, F. H., Jr. and Diamond, L. K.: Erythroblastosis fetalis. *N. Engl. J. Med.* 257:659, 1957.
3. Altwater, J., *et al.*: Sickling of erythrocytes in a patient with thalassemia-hemoglobin I disease. *N. Engl. J. Med.* 263:1215, 1960.
4. Armata, J., *et al.*: Thrombocytosis in acute leukemia. *Pol. med. Sci. His.* 14:55, 1971.
5. Athens, J. W.: Leukocyte physiology (in Medical News). *J.A.M.A.* 198:38, 1966.
6. Baar, H. S.: *Disorders of Blood and Blood-forming Organs in Childhood.* Hafner, New York, 1963.
7. Bacus, J. W.: Erythrocyte morphology and centrifugal "spinner" blood film preparations. *J. Histochem. Cytochem.* 22:506, 1974.
8. Bainton, D. F. and Finch, C. A.: The diagnosis of iron deficiency anemia. *Am. J. Med.* 37:62, 1964.
9. Bannerman, R. M. and Renwick, J. A.: The hereditary elliptocytoses; clinical and linkage data. *Ann. Hum. Genet* 26:23, 1962.
10. Bassen, F. A. and Kornzweig, A. L.: Malformation of the erythrocytes in a case of atypical retinitis pigmentosa. *Blood* 5:381, 1950.
11. Beck, W. S., editor: *Hematology.* Harvard Pathophysiology Series, Vol. I. MIT Press, Cambridge, MA, 1973.
12. Begemann, N. H. and Campagne, A. V. L.: Homozygous form of Pelger-Huet nuclear anomaly in man. *Acta Haematol.* 7:295, 1952.
13. Bentley, H. P., *et al.*: Eosinophilic leukemia. *Am. J. Med.* 30:340, 1961.
14. Benvenisti, D. S. and Ultmann, J. E.: Eosinophilic leukemia. Report of five cases and review of the literature. *Ann. Intern. med.* 7:731, 1969.
15. Benz, E. J., Jr. and Forget, B. G.: The biosynthesis of hemoglobin. *Semin. Hematol.* 11:463, 1974.
16. Berman, L., *et al.*: The blood and bone marrow in patients with cirrhosis of the liver. *Blood* 4:511, 1949.
17. Bessis, M. C. and Breton-Gorius, J.: Iron particles in normal erythroblasts and in pathologic erythrocytes. *J. Biophys. Biochem. Cytol.* 3:503, 1957.
18. Bessis, M. C. and Breton-Gorius, J.: Iron metabolism in the bone marrow as seen by electron microscopy. *Blood* 14:423, 1959; 19:635, 1962; *Rev. Hemat.* 14:165, 1959.
19. Bingham, J.: The macrocytosis of liver disease. *Blood* 14:694, 1959; 15;244, 1960.
20. Boggs, D. R., *et al.*: The acute leukemias. *Medicine (Baltimore)* 41:163, 1962.
21. Bookchin, R. M., *et al.*: Hemoglobin C$_{Harlem}$: A sickling variant containing amino acid substitutions in two residues of the α-polypeptide chain. *Biochem. Biophys. Res. Commun.* 23:122, 1966.
22. Boseila, A.: Hormonal influence on blood and tissue basophilic granulocytes. *Ann. N.Y. Acad. Sci.* 103:394, 1963.
23. Boveri, R. M.: The errors in the differential blood count comparison of the slide and coverglass methods. *Guy's Hosp. Rep.* 89:112, 1939.
24. Bowman, W. D., Jr.: Abnormal (ringed) sideroblasts in various hematologic and non-hematologic disorders. *Blood* 18:662, 1961.
25. Brain, M. C.: Microangiopathic hemolytic anemia. *N. Engl. J. Med.* 281:833, 1969.
26. Brain, M. C.: Microangiopathic hemolytic anemia. *Br. J. Haematol.* 23(suppl):45, 1972.
27. Brain, M. C., Dacie, J. V., and Hourihance, D. O. D.: Microangiopathic hemolytic anemia. The possible role of vascular lesions in pathogenesis. *Br. J. Haematol.* 8:358, 1962.
28. Brunning, R. D.: Morphologic alteration in nucleated blood and marrow cells in genetic disorders. *Hum. Pathol.* 1: p. 103, No. I, March, 1970.
29. Bull, B. S. and Kuhn, I. N.: The production of schistocytes by fibrin strands (a scanning electron microscope study). *Blood* 35:99–124, 1970.
30. Burns, C. P., *et al.*: Biochemical, morphological and immunological observations of leukemic reticulo-endotheliosis. *Cancer Res.* 33:1615, 1973.

31. Cartwright, G. E.: *Diagnostic Laboratory Hematology*, 4th ed. Grune & Stratton, New York, 1968.

32. Chandra, R. K. and Bhakoo, O. N.: Leuco-erythroblastic (leukaemoid) reaction in infants and children. *Indian J. Pediat.* 2:411, 1965.

33. Charache, S. and Waugh, D.: Pathogenesis of hemolytic anemia in homozygous hemoglobin C disease. *J. Clin. Invest.* 46:1795, 1967.

34. Chediak, M. M.: Nouvelle anomalie leucocytaire de caractere constitutionnel et familial. *Rev. Haematol.* 7:362, 1952.

35. Clough, P. W.: Monocytic leukemia. *Bull. Johns Hopkins Hosp.* 51:148, 1932.

36. Colman, R. W. and Shein, H. M.: Leukemoid reaction, hyperuricemia and severe hyperpyrexia complicating a fatal case of acute fatty liver of the alcoholic. *Ann. Intern. Med.* 57:110, 1962.

37. Crossen, P. E., *et al.*: The Sézary syndrome. Cytogenetic studies and identification of the Sézary cell as an abnormal lymphocyte. *Am. J. Med.* 50:24, 1971.

38. Cudkowicz, G., Bennett, M., and Shearer, G. M.: Pluripotent stem cell function of the mouse marrow lymphocyte. *Science* 144:866, 1964.

39. Cutting, H. O., McHugh, W. J., Conrad, F. G., and Marlowe, A. A.: Autosomal dominant hemolytic anemia characterized by ovalocytosis. *Am. J. Med.* 39:21, 1965.

40. Dacie, J. V. and Lewis, S. M.: *Practical Hematology.* Grune & Stratton Inc., New York, 1968.

41. Daland, G. A., *et al.*: Hematologic observations in bacterial endocarditis. *J. Lab. Clin. Med.* 48:827, 1956.

42. Dameschek, W.: Acute monocytic (histiocytic) leukemia: Review of literature and case reports. *Arch. Intern. Med.* 46:718, 1930.

43. Dameschek, W.: Chronic lymphocytic leukemia—An accumulative disease of immunologically incompetent lymphocytes. *Blood* 29:566, 1967.

44. Davidsohn, I. and Henry, J. B.: *Clinical Diagnosis Laboratory Methods*, 15th ed. W. B. Saunders Co., Philadelphia, 1974.

45. Davidsohn, W. M. and Smith, D. R.: A morphologic sex difference in the polymorphic leukocytes. *Br. Med. J.* 2:6, 1954.

46. Davidsohn, W. M., *et al.*: The Pelger-Huet anomaly: Investigation of family "A." *Ann. Hum. Genet.* 19:1, 1954.

47. Diggs, L. W., *et al.*: Intraerythrocytic crystals in a white patient with hemoglobin C in the absence of other types of hemoglobin. *Blood* 9:1172, 1954.

48. Diggs, L. W. and Bell, A.: *Morphology of Human Blood Cells.* Sponsored by Council on Hematology, Commission on Continuing Education, American Society of Clinical Pathology, 1965.

49. Discombe, G.: L'origine des corps de Howell-Jolly et des anneaux de Cabot. *Sangre* 29:262, 1948.

50. Dohle, H.: Leukocyteneinschluesse bei Scharlach. *Zentralbl. Bakteriol.* 61:63, 1911.

51. Donhauser, J. L.: The human spleen as an haematopoietic organ, as exemplified in a case of splenomegaly with sclerosis of the bone marrow. *J. Exp. Med.* 10:559, 1908.

52. Donohugh, D. L.: Eosinophils and eosinophilia. *Calif. Med.* 104:521, 1966.

53. Dorr, A. D. and Moloney, W. C.: Acquired pseudo-Pelger-Huet anomaly of granulocytic leukocytes. *N. Engl. J. Med.* 261:742, 1959.

54. Douglas, A. S. and Dacie, J. V.: The incidence and significance of iron-containing granules in human erythrocytes and their precursors. *J. Clin. Pathol.* 6:307, 1953.

55. Downey, H. and MacKinlay, C. A.: Acute lymphadenosis compared with acute lymphatic leukemia. *Arch. Intern. Med.* 32:82, 1923.

56. Dubos, R. J. and Hirsch, J. G.: *Bacterial and Mycotic Infections of Man*, 4th ed. J. B. Lippincott Co., Philadelphia, 1965.

57. Dutcher, T. F.: Bands, polys, and atypical lymphs—One more time! Lab. Med. **6**, No. 11, p. 20, Nov. 1975.

58. Ewald, O.: Die leukamische reticuloendotheliose. *Dtsch. Arch. Kinderheilkd. Med.* 142:222, 1923.

59. Finch, S. C.: *Infectious Mononucleosis.* Blackwell Scientific Publications, Oxford, 1969.

60. Fischer, R., *et al.*: Der cytochemisch nachweis von naphthol-AS-D-chloroacetat-esterase in Auerstabchen. *Klin. Wochenschr.* 44:401, 1966.

61. Freeman, A. I. and Journey, L. J.: Ultrastructural studies on monocytic leukemia. *Br. J. Haematol.* 20:225, 1971.

62. Freeman, J. A.: Origin of Auer bodies. *Blood* 27:499, 1966.

63. Garrey, W. E. and Bryan, W. R.: Variations in white blood counts. *Physiol. Rev.* 15:597, 1935.

64. Gilmer, P. R. and Koepke, J. A.: The reticulocyte: An approach to definition. *Am. J. Clin. Pathol.* 66:263, 1976.

65. Goldberg, A. F.: Acid phosphatase activity in Auer bodies. *Blood* 24:305, 1964.

66. Gordin, R.: Toxic granulation in leukocytes. *Acta Med. Scand.* Suppl. 270, 1952.

67. Gordon, A. S.: Quantitative nature of the red cell response to a single bleeding. *Proc. Soc. Exp. Biol. Med.* 31:563, 1934.

68. Griffin, H.: Persistent eosinophilia with hyperleukocytosis and splenomegaly. *Am. J. Med. Sci.* 158:618, 1919.

69. Groover, R. V., *et al.*: The genetic mucopolysaccharidoses. *Semin. Hemat.* 9:371, 1972.

70. Gruneberg, H.: Siderocytes: A new kind of erythrocytes. *Nature* 148:114, 1941a.

71. Gruneberg, H.: Siderocytes in man. *Nature* 148:469, 1941b.

72. Hahn, E. V.: Sickle cell (drepanocytic) anemia with a report of a second case successfully treated by a splenectomy and further observations on the mechanism of sickle cell formation. *Am. J. Med. Sci.* 175–206, 1928.

73. Ham, T. H., *et al.*: Studies on the destruction of red blood cells. IV. *Blood* 3:373, 1948.

74. Harada, N.: Histochemical studies on Auer body. *Nagoya J. Med. Sci.* 14:129, 1951.

75. Hardy, W. R. and Anderson, R. E.: The hypereosinophilic syndromes. *Ann. Intern. Med.* 68:1220, 1968.

76. Harris, J. W. and Kellermeyer, R. W.: *The Red Cell, Production, Metabolism, Destruction: Normal and Abnormal.* Harvard University Press, Cambridge, MA, 1970.

77. Hartsock, R. J.: Fundamental teachings in hematology, in *Listen, Look and Learn Audiovisual Study Unit for the Medical Laboratory,* Vol. III, Coagulation, Hematology, 1972.

78. Hayhoe, F. G. J., Quaglino, D., and Doll, R.: The cytology and cytochemistry of acute leukemias: A study of 104 cases. *M.R.C. Special Reports Series,* No. 304. H. M. Stationery Office, London, 1964.

79. Hegglin, R.: Über eine besondereform gliechzeitiger konstitutioneller Veranderungen der Neutrophilen und Thrombozyten (Konstitutionelle polyphile Reifungsstorung)! Arch. Klaus-Stify. Vererb-Forsch., Zurich, 20:1, 1945a.

80. Hegglin, R.: Gleichzeitige konstitutionelle Veranderungen an Neutrophilen und Thrombozyten! *Helv. Med. Acta* 12:439, 1945b.

81. Heilmeyer, L.: Blutfarbstoff Wechselstudien. *Dtsch. Arch. Klin. Med.* 171:123, 1931.

82. *Hematology Check Sample No. 45, Basophilic Leukemia.* Check Sample Program, Commission on Continuing Education, American Society of Clinical Pathologists, Chicago, 1970.

83. Hickling, R. A.: The monocytes in pneumonia—A clinical and hematologic study. *Arch. Intern. Med.* 40:594, 1927.

84. Higashi, O.: Congenital abnormality of peroxidase granules—A case of "congenital gigantism of peroxidase granules," preliminary report. *Tohoku J. Exp. Med.* 58:246, 1953; 59:315, 1954.

85. Hillman, R. S. and Finch, C. A.: *Red Cell Manual,* 4th Ed. F. A. Davis Co., Philadelphia, 1974.

86. Hilts, S. V. and Shaw, C. C.: Leukemoid blood reactions. *N. Engl. J. Med.* 249:434, 1953.

87. Hittmair, A.: Beitrayzur basophilen leukamie. *Schweiz Med. Wochenschr.,* 90, 938, 1960.

88. Hoagland, R. J.: Infectious mononucleosis. *Am. J. Med.* 13:158, 1952; *Ann. Intern. Med.* 43:1019, 1955; *Am. J. Med. Sci.* 232:252, 1956, 240:21, 1960; *Blood* 16:1045, 1960.

89. Horsfall, F. L. and Tamm, I.: *Viral and Rickettsial Infections of Man,* 4th ed. J. B. Lippincott Co., Philadelphia, 1965.

90. Huet, G. J.: Familial anomaly of leukocytes. *Discuss. Med. Tijdschr. Geneesk.* 75:5956, 1931.

91. Ingram, V. M.: A specific chemical difference between the globins of normal human and sickle cell anemia haemoglobin. *Nature* 178:792, 1956. *Conference on Hemoglobin.* National Academy of Sciences 1958, Publication 557.

92. Ingram, V. M.: *The Hemoglobins in Genetics and Evolution.* Columbia University Press, New York, 1963.

93. Itoga, T. and Laszlo, J.: Dohle bodies and other granulocytic alterations with cyclophosphamide. *Blood* 20:668, 1962.

94. Jacob, H. S.: Abnormalities in the physiology of the erythrocyte's membrane in hereditary spherocytosis. *Am. J. Med.* 41:734, 1966.

95. Jacobson, L. B., *et al.*: Clinical and immunologic features of transient cold agglutinin hemolytic anemia. *Am. J. Med.* 54:514, 1973.

96. Jandl, J. H.: Hereditary spherocytosis, in E. Beutler, *Hereditary Disorders of Erythrocyte Metabolism,* edited by Grune & Stratton, New York, 1968.

97. Jensen, W. N. and Moreno, G.: Les ribosomes et les ponctuations basophiles des erythrocytes dans l'intoxication par le ploml. *C. R. Acad. Sci. (Paris)* 258:3596, 1964.

98. Jensen, W. N., Moreno, G., and Bessis, M.: An electron microscopic description of basophilic stippling in red blood cells. *Blood* 25:933, 1965.

99. Kass, L.: Origin and composition of Cabot ring in pernicious anemia. *Am. J. Clin. Pathol.* 64: p. 554, No. 1, July, 1975.

100. Koyama, S.: Studies on the Howell-Jolly body. *Acta Hematol. Japan* 23:20, 1960.

101. Krumblar, E. B.: Leukemoid blood pictures in various clinical conditions. *Am. J. Med. Sci.* 172:519, 1926.

102. Kunkel, H. G., *et al.*: Observations on the minor basic hemoglobin components in the blood of normal individuals and patients with thalassemia. *J. Clin. Invest.* 36:615, 1957.

103. Kyle, R. A. and Pease, G. L.: Basophilic leukemia. *Arch. Intern. Med.* 118:205, 1966.

104. Leavell, B. S. and Thorup, O. A., Jr.: *Fundamentals of Hematology*, 4th ed. W. B. Saunders Co., Philadelphia, 1976.

105. Lecks, H. I. and Kravis, L.: The allergist and the eosinophil. *Pediatr. Clin. N. Am.* 16:125, 1969.

106. Lee, R. E. and Ellis, L. D.: The storage cells of chronic myelogenous leukemia. *Lab. Invest.* 24:261, 1971.

107. Lessin, L. S.: Membrane ultrastructure of normal sickled and Heinz body erythrocytes by freeze etching, in *Red Cell Shape*, edited by M. Bessis, R. Weed, and P. LeBland. Springer-Verlag, New York, 1973.

108. Levinson, S. A. and MacFate, R. P.: *Clinical Laboratory Diagnosis*, 6th ed. Lea & Febiger, Philadelphia 1961.

109. Lie-Injo, L. E.: Hemoglobin Bart's and the sickling phenomenon. *Nature* 191:1314, 1961.

110. Lipson, R. L., *et al.*: The post-splenectomy blood picture. *Am. J. Clin. Pathol.* 32:526, 1959.

111. Lubrano, G. J., *et al.*: The analysis of some commercial dyes and Romanowsky stains by high-performance liquid chromatography. *Stain Technol.* 52: p. 13, No. 1, 1977.

112. Lutzner, M. and Jordan, H. W.: The ultrastructure of an abnormal cell in Sezary syndrome. *Blood* 31:719, 1968.

113. MacGregor, R. G., *et al.*: The differential leucocyte count. *J. Pathol.* 51:337, 1940.

114. MacLean, N. and Edin, M. B.: The drumsticks of polymorphonuclear leukocytes in sex-chromosome abnormalities. *Lancet* 1:1154, 1962.

115. Maldonado, J. E. and Hanlon, D. G.: Monocytosis: A current appraisal. *Mayo Clinic Proc.* 40:248, 1965.

116. Maldonado, N. I., *et al.*: Case report: Autoimmune hemolytic anemia in chronic myelogenous leukemia. *Blood* 30:518, 1967.

117. Marsh, J. C.: Analysis of one hundred and six patients with chronic myelogenous leukemia examined in the University of Utah hematology clinic from 1944 to 1963. (unpublished).

118. Mathe, G., *et al.*: Subdivision of classical varieties of acute lymphocytic leukemia: A correlation with prognosis and cure expectancy. *Eur. J. Clin. Biol. Res.* 16:554, 1971.

119. May, R.: "Leukocyteneinschlusse." *Dtsch. Arch. Klin. Med.* 96:1, 1909.

120. McCall, C. E., *et al.*: Lysosomal and ultrastructural changes in human "toxic" neutrophils during bacterial infection. *J. Exp. Med.* 129:267, 1969; *J. Infect. Dis.* 124:68, 1971; 127:26, 1973.

121. McDonald, G. A., Dodds, T. C., and Cruickshank, B.: *Atlas of Hematology*, 3rd ed. Baltimore, Williams & Wilkins, 1970.

122. McKee, L. C., *et al.*: Experimental iron deficiency in the rat. *Br. J. Haematol.* 14:87, 1968.

123. Megla, G. K.: Automatic blood film preparation by rheologically controlled spinning. *Am. J. Med. Technol.* 42:3–14, No. 9, Sept. 1976.

124. Milhorat, A. T., Small, S. M., and Diethelm, O.: Leukocytosis during various emotional states. *Arch. Neurol. Psychiatry* 47:779, 1942.

125. Miller, S. E., *et al.*: *A Textbook of Clinical Pathology*, 7th ed. Williams & Wilkins, Baltimore, 1966.

126. Mollin, D. L.: Sideroblasts and sideroblastic anemia. *Br. J. Haematol.* 11:41, 1965.

127. Mollison, P. L.: *Blood Transfusion in Clinical Medicine*, 5th ed. Blackwell Scientific Publications, Oxford, 1972.

128. Nachtsheim, H.: The Pelger anomaly in man and rabbit. A Mendelian character of the nuclei of the leukocytes. *J. Hered.* 41:131, 1950.

129. Nelson, D. A. and Davey, F. R.: Leukocyte esterase, in *Hematology*, 2nd ed., edited by W. J. Williams, *et al.* McGraw-Hill Book Co., New York, 1976.

130. Nourbakhsh, M., *et al.*: An evaluation of blood smears made by a new method using a spinner and diluted blood. *Am. J. Clin. Pathol.* 70: No. 6, Dec. 1978.

131. Oski, F. A. and Naumann, J. L.: Hematologic problems in the newborn, see Erythroblastosis fetalis, *Major Problems in Clinical Pediatrics*, 4:176, 1972.

132. Ozer, F. L. and Mills, G. L.: Elliptocytosis with hemolytic anemia. *Br. J. Haematol.* 10:468, 1964.

133. Page, L. B. and Culver, P. J.: *A Syllabus of Laboratory Examinations in Clinical Diagnosis*. Harvard University Press, Cambridge, MA, 1966.

134. Pappenheimer, A. M., *et al.*: Anemia associated with unidentified erythrocytic inclusions after splenectomy. *Q. J. Med. N. S.* 14:75, 1945.

135. Pelger, K.: Demonstratie van een paar Zeldzaam voorkomende typen van bloedlichaampjes en bespreking der patienten. *Discuss. Med. Tijdschr. Geneesk.* 72:1178, 1928.

136. Perkins, H. A., *et al.*: Hemostatic defects in dysproteinemias. *Blood* 35:695, 1970.

137. Petzel, G. and Undritz, E.: Ein Teiltrager der Pelger-Huetschen Blutkorperchenanomalie mit heterozygoten Pelgerzellen von typ Stodmeister. *Fol. Haematol.* 1:268, 1957.
138. Pierce, L. E., *et al.*: A new hemoglobin variant with sickling properties. *N. Engl. J. Med.* 268:862, 1963.
139. Preston, K. and Ingram, M.: Automatic analysis of blood cells. *Sci. Am.* 223: No. 5, 76, Nov. 1970.
140. Preston, K., Norgren, P. E., and Bossung, J.: Methods of preparing blood smears. *U.S. Patent No. 3,577,267*, May, 1971.
141. Quatrin, N., *et al.*: Basophile leukamien. *Blut* 5:166, 1959.
142. Raphael, S. S.: *Lynch's Medical Laboratory Technology*, 3rd ed. W. B. Saunders Co., Philadelphia, 1976.
143. Ravel, R. and Bassart, J. A.: Platelet satellitosis and phagocytosis by leukocytes. *Lab. Med.* 5:41–42, No. 6, June, 1974.
144. Rebuck, J. W.: *Hematology Check Sample No. 39, Agnogenic Myeloid Metaplasia.* Check Sample Program, Commission on Continuing Education, American Society of Clinical Pathologists, Chicago, 1970.
145. Reilly, W. A.: The granules in the leukocytes in gargoylism. *Am. J. Dis. Child.* 62:489, 1941.
146. Reisner, E. G., Jr.: Morphology of erythrocytes in erythroblastosis fetalis. *Arch. Intern. Med.* 71:230, 1943.
147. Rey, J. J. and Wolf, P. L.: Extreme leukocytosis in accidental electric shock. *Lancet* 1:18, 1968.
148. Rifkind, R. A.: Heinz body anemia: An ultrastructural study II, red cell sequestration and destruction. *Blood* 26:433, 1965.
149. Rifkind, R. A. and Danon, D.: Heinz body anemia: An ultrastructure study. I. Heinz body formation. *Blood* 25:885, 1965.
150. Roger, C. H.: Blood sample preparation for automated differential systems. *Am. J. Med. Technol.* 39:435–442, No. 11, Nov. 1973.
151. Rosenthal, R. L.: Acute promyelocytic leukemia associated with hypofibrinogenemia. *Blood* 21:495, 1963.
152. Rubenberg, M. L., *et al.*: Microangiopathic hemolytic anemia: The experimental induction of hemolysis and red blood cell fragmentation by defibrination *in vivo. Br. J. Haematol.* 14:627, 1968.
153. Salt, H. B., *et al.*: On having no beta-lipoprotein. A syndrome comprising a beta-lipoproteinemia, acanthocytosis and steatorrhea. *Lancet* 2:325, 1960.
154. Schneider, R. G., *et al.*: Hemoglobin I in an American Negro family: Structural and hematologic studies. *J. Lab. Clin. Med.* 68:940, 1966.
155. Schrek, R. and Donnelly, W. J.: "Hairy" cells in blood in lymphoreticular neoplastic disease and "flagellated" cells of normal lymph nodes. *Blood* 27:199, 1966.
156. Schubothe, H.: The cold hemagglutinin disease. *Semin. Hematol.* 3:27, 1966.
157. Schwartz, J.: Adherence and phagocytosis of erythrocytes by *in vitro* cultured macrophages. *J. Reticuloendothel. Soc.* 4:109, 1967; 9:528, 1971.
158. Seaman, A. J. and Starr, A.: Febrile postcardiotomy lymphocytic splenomegaly. *Ann. Surg.* 145:956, 1962.
159. Sézary, A.: La reticulose maligne leucemique a histio-monocytes monstreux et a forme d'erythrodermie eodemateuse et pigmentie. *Ann. Derm. Syph.* 9:5, 1949.
160. Sheehy, T. W. and Berman, A.: The anemia of cirrhosis. *J. Lab. Clin. Med.* 56:72, 1960.
161. Sheets, R. F., *et al.*: Erythroleukemia (di Guglielmo's syndrome). *Arch. Intern. Med.* 111:295, 1963.
162. Shelley, W. B.: The circulating basophil as indication of hypersensitivity in man. *Arch. Dermatol.* 88:759, 1963.
163. Silbergeit, A.: A study of platelet-leukocyte aggregation in coronary thrombosis and cerebral thrombosis. *Thromb. Diath. Haemorr.*, Suppl. 42, 155, 1970.
164. Simmons, A.: *Technical Hematology*, 2nd ed. J. B. Lippincott Co., Philadelphia, 1976.
165. Simon, E. R. and Ways, P.: Incubation hemolysis and red blood cell metabolism in acanthocytosis. *J. Clin. Invest.* 43:1311, 1964.
166. Sinay, H. and O'Connor, B.: Manual peripheral blood differential cell counting procedure. Yale-New Haven Hospital Hematology Laboratory, 1967 (unpublished).
167. Skendzel, L. P. and Hoffman, G. C.: The Pelger anomaly of leukocytes; forty-one cases in seven families. *Am. J. Clin. Pathol.* 37:294, 1962.
168. Smith, D. R.: A syndrome resembling infectious mononucleosis after open heart surgery. *Br. Med. J.* 1:945, 1964.
169. Smith, E. W. and Conley, C. L.: Filter paper electrophoresis of human hemoglobins with special reference to the incidence and clinical significance of hemoglobin C. *Johns Hopkins Med. J.* 93:94, 1953.
170. Stuart, A. E., *et al.*: A biological test for injury to the human red cell. *Vox Sang.* 13:270, 1967; *J. Reticuloendothel. Soc.* 4:109, 1967; 9:528, 1971.

171. Trubowitz, S., Masek, B., and Frasca, J. M.: Leukemic reticuloendothelioses. *Blood* 38:288, 1971.
172. Tullis, J. L.: A case of leukocytosis in diabetes acidosis; effects of experimental hypertonia on circulating leukocytes. *J. Clin. Invest.* 26:1098, 1947.
173. Undritz, E.: Les malformations hereditaires des elements figures du sang. *Sangre* 25:296, 1954.
174. Undritz, E., editor: *Sandoz Atlas of Hematology*, 2nd ed. Sandoz Ltd., Basle, Switzerland, 1973.
175. Venkatachalam, M. A., Jones, D. B., and Nelson, D. A.: Microangiopathic hemolytic anemia in rats with malignant hypertension. *Blood* 32:278, 1968.
176. Weatherall, D. J.: Biochemical phenotypes of thalassemia in the American Negro population. *Ann. N. Y. Acad. Sci.* 119:450, 1964.
177. Weatherall, D. J. and Clegg, J. B.: *The Thalassemia Syndromes*, 2nd ed. Blackwell Scientific Publications, Oxford, 1972.
178. Weed, R. I., *et al.*: Metabolic dependence of red cell deformability. *J. Clin. Invest.* 48:795, 1969.
179. Weiner, W. and Topley, E.: Dohle bodies in leukocytes of patients with burns. *J. Clin. Pathol.* 8:324, 1955.
180. Wenk, R. E.: Comparison of five methods for preparing blood smear. *Am. J. Med. Technol.* 42:71–78, No. 3, March, 1976.
181. Wheby, M. S., *et al.*: Homozygous hemoglobin C disease in siblings; further comment on intraerythrocytic crystals. *Blood* 11:266, 1956.
182. Wiley, J. S., *et al.*: Characteristics of the membrane defect in hereditary stomatocytosis syndrome. *Blood* 46:337, 1975.
183. Williams, W. J., *et al.*: *Hematology*, 1st ed. McGraw-Hill Book Co., New York, 1972.
184. Williams, W. J., *et al.*: *Hematology*, 2nd ed. McGraw-Hill Book Co., New York, 1976.
185. Wintrobe, M. M.: *Clinical Hematology*, 5th ed. Lea & Febiger, Philadelphia, 1961.
186. Wintrobe, M. M.: *Clinical Hematology*, 6th ed. Lea & Febiger, Philadelphia, 1967.
187. Wintrobe, M. M., *et al.*: *Clinical Hematology*, 7th ed. Lea & Febiger, Philadelphia, 1974.
188. Witts, L. J., *et al.*: Chronic granulocytic leukemia: Comparison of radiotherapy and busulphan therapy. Report of the Medical Research Council's Working Party for Therapeutic Trials in Leukemia. *Br. Med. J.* 1:201, 1968.
189. Zinkham, W. H. and Diamond, L. K.: In vitro erythrophagocytosis in acquired hemolytic anemia. *Blood* 7:592, 1952.
190. Zittoun, R.: Subacute and chronic myelo-monocytic leukemia: A distinct hematological entity. *Br. J. Haematol.* 32:1, 1976.